Beyond Borders—Tackling Neglected Tropical Viral Diseases

Beyond Borders—Tackling Neglected Tropical Viral Diseases

Guest Editor

Jelena Prpić

MDPI

Basel • Beijing • Wuhan • Barcelona • Belgrade • Novi Sad • Cluj • Manchester

Guest Editor
Jelena Prpić
Croatian Veterinary Institute
Zagreb
Croatia

Editorial Office
MDPI AG
Grosspeteranlage 5
4052 Basel, Switzerland

This is a reprint of the Special Issue, published open access by the journal *Tropical Medicine and Infectious Disease* (ISSN 2414-6366), freely accessible at: https://www.mdpi.com/journal/tropicalmed/special_issues/4E5684799O.

For citation purposes, cite each article independently as indicated on the article page online and as indicated below:

Lastname, A.A.; Lastname, B.B. Article Title. *Journal Name* **Year**, *Volume Number*, Page Range.

ISBN 978-3-7258-6710-3 (Hbk)
ISBN 978-3-7258-6711-0 (PDF)
https://doi.org/10.3390/books978-3-7258-6711-0

Contents

About the Editor

Jelena Prpić

Jelena Prpić is a Scientific Associate at the Croatian Veterinary Institute in Zagreb, specializing in veterinary virology, zoonotic infections, and the molecular epidemiology of emerging and neglected viral diseases. Her research focuses on hepatitis E virus, arboviruses, and viral pathogens at the animal–human interface, with a strong emphasis on the One Health approach. She has contributed to numerous national and international research projects, including studies on HEV epidemiology, tick-borne pathogens, neuroinvasive arboviruses, and coordinated disease surveillance systems. She is an active member of the COST Action ONWARD, dedicated to establishing a European network for zoonotic hepevirus research and harmonized surveillance. Her scientific achievements include multiple peer-reviewed publications, editorial work for Special Issues on emerging viral zoonoses, and extensive experience in molecular diagnostics, phylogenetic analysis, and wildlife disease surveillance. Through her interdisciplinary work, she aims to strengthen our understanding of zoonotic viral threats and support evidence-based public health and veterinary strategies in Croatia and beyond.

Preface

Viral neglected tropical diseases continue to evolve in complexity and reach, increasingly affecting regions far beyond their traditional boundaries. This Special Issue was assembled to address these shifting dynamics and to showcase interdisciplinary research that advances early detection, vector surveillance, diagnostic innovation, and clinical insight. The articles collected here underscore the importance of community engagement, cross-border collaboration, and resilient public health systems in mitigating the growing burden of arboviral diseases. I extend my sincere appreciation to all contributing authors and reviewers whose work enriches our understanding and strengthens the global response to these persistent threats.

Jelena Prpić
Guest Editor

Tropical Medicine and Infectious Disease

MDPI

Editorial

Beyond Borders—Tackling Neglected Tropical Viral Diseases

Jelena Prpić

Croatian Veterinary Institute, 10000 Zagreb, Croatia; balatinec@veinst.hr

Neglected tropical diseases (NTDs) comprise a diverse group of infections that disproportionately affect impoverished populations in tropical and subtropical regions. Among them, viral NTDs, including dengue, Zika, chikungunya, yellow fever, West Nile virus, Oropouche virus, and other emerging arboviruses, represent a growing global health concern due to their expanding geographic distribution, increasing incidence, and complex interactions with environmental and socioeconomic factors [1–3]. More than one hundred arboviruses are known to infect humans, and many continue to emerge or re-emerge as ecological and climatic conditions shift. According to the World Health Organization (WHO), nearly 3.9 billion people now live in areas at risk for *Aedes*-borne arboviral infections, and the frequency and magnitude of outbreaks have increased markedly over the past decade, driven by climate variability, rapid urbanization, and intensified human mobility [2–4].

The WHO's Global Arbovirus Initiative underscores the urgency of coordinated global action, emphasizing that arboviruses such as dengue, Zika, chikungunya, and yellow fever are expanding into new ecological niches and placing unprecedented strain on public health systems. Climate change is accelerating vector expansion into temperate regions, including parts of Europe, where *Aedes albopictus* and *Aedes aegypti* have become increasingly established [5]. These shifts are reshaping arboviral transmission dynamics and challenging traditional assumptions about the geographic limits of tropical viral diseases.

Beyond environmental drivers, structural vulnerabilities, including inadequate vector control, limited access to diagnostics, fragile health systems, and insufficient community engagement, continue to exacerbate the burden of viral NTDs [3,4]. Surveillance gaps allow silent transmission to persist for years before major outbreaks are detected, particularly in low-resource settings. Although advances in biomedical research have improved diagnostic and surveillance capacities, many endemic regions still lack the laboratory infrastructure needed for timely detection and response. Interdisciplinary research increasingly highlights the importance of integrating community-based strategies with scientific innovation to strengthen outbreak preparedness and improve public health outcomes.

Addressing these challenges requires coordinated, cross-border, and interdisciplinary approaches that integrate epidemiology, vector biology, diagnostics, clinical research, and community engagement. As global mobility intensifies and climate change accelerates, the need for adaptive and collaborative public health responses has never been greater.

In this Special Issue of Tropical Medicine and Infectious Diseases, "Beyond Borders—Tackling Neglected Tropical Viral Diseases", we invited contributions that explore innovative strategies, research advances, and collaborative efforts aimed at understanding and controlling neglected tropical viral diseases. Eight articles, spanning epidemiological analyses, diagnostic innovation, seroprevalence studies, systematic reviews, and immunological insights, were published.

Costa-Ribeiro et al. assessed the impact of mass dengue vaccination on disease incidence in Paraná, Brazil, using an interrupted time series approach [6]. Their findings highlight the potential of large-scale immunization programs to reduce dengue burden, while also emphasizing the importance of continuous monitoring and adaptive public health strategies.

Reigoto et al. explored the use of limited near-infrared spectroscopy data combined with machine learning to detect Zika virus infection in *Aedes aegypti* mosquitoes [7]. This innovative vector-based diagnostic approach demonstrates the feasibility of rapid, non-destructive surveillance tools, particularly valuable in resource-limited settings.

Chandrasena et al. conducted a systematic review and meta-analysis of dengue-related knowledge, attitudes, and practices (KAPs) among the general public in Sri Lanka from 2000 to 2023 [8]. Their synthesis reveals persistent gaps in community awareness and preventive behaviors, underscoring the need for sustained, culturally tailored health education initiatives.

To et al. evaluated baseline IgG seroprevalence of multiple arboviruses in Liberia using a multiplex immunoassay [9]. Their findings demonstrate widespread exposure to several arboviruses, highlighting the silent circulation of these pathogens and the need for integrated serological surveillance in West Africa.

Amaral et al. performed a systematic review and meta-analysis examining the association between chikungunya fever and rheumatoid arthritis [10]. Their results suggest that chikungunya infection may trigger or exacerbate chronic inflammatory joint disease, emphasizing the long-term clinical consequences of arboviral infections.

Melebari et al. characterized dengue virus serotypes among patients presenting with dengue fever in Makkah, Saudi Arabia [11]. Their identification of multiple co-circulating serotypes provides essential information for anticipating outbreaks and guiding clinical and public health preparedness in a region marked by intense international travel.

He et al. reviewed the mechanisms by which bunyaviruses suppress interferon responses and summarized current antiviral strategies [12]. Their work highlights the sophisticated immune evasion tactics of bunyaviruses and identifies potential therapeutic targets.

Finally, Ríos-Bracamontes et al. analyzed national surveillance data from Mexico (2020–2024) to identify factors associated with in-hospital dengue mortality [13]. Their findings provide critical insights into clinical predictors of severe disease and underscore the importance of early recognition and optimized case management.

The articles presented in this Special Issue collectively underscore that neglected tropical viral diseases remain among the most dynamic and challenging threats to global health. Despite decades of scientific progress, the persistent and often widening gaps in surveillance, diagnostics, vector control, and clinical management reveal how deeply these diseases are intertwined with structural inequities. The research showcased here demonstrates that scientific innovation alone is not sufficient; rather, it must be paired with sustained investment in public health infrastructure, community engagement, and international cooperation.

A recurring theme across the contributions is the importance of early detection and rapid response. Whether through innovative vector-based diagnostic tools, multiplex serological assays, or improved epidemiological modeling, the ability to identify outbreaks before they escalate is essential. Strengthening laboratory capacity and integrating novel technologies into routine surveillance can help countries detect silent transmission, monitor serotype shifts, and anticipate severe disease outcomes.

Another critical insight emerging from this Special Issue is the long-term clinical and societal impact of arboviral infections. Studies examining chronic sequelae, such as chikungunya-associated inflammatory disease, highlight the need for long-term patient follow-up and improved clinical guidelines. These findings challenge the misconception

 https://doi.org/10.3390/tropicalmed11010029

that arboviral infections are self-limiting and emphasize the importance of integrating post-acute care into national health strategies.

The contributions also reinforce the central role of community knowledge, behavior, and trust in shaping outbreak trajectories. Persistent gaps in public awareness, as documented in Sri Lanka and other endemic regions, demonstrate that effective vector control and prevention strategies depend on culturally informed, community-centered approaches. Public health messaging must be continuous, context-specific, and responsive to local perceptions and barriers.

Importantly, the Special Issue highlights how global forces, climate change, urbanization, migration, and international travel are reshaping arboviral ecology. These forces transcend national borders, making unilateral approaches insufficient. Cross-border data sharing, harmonized surveillance systems, and coordinated vector control strategies are essential to prevent the spread of arboviruses into new regions and to mitigate the impact of outbreaks in highly interconnected societies.

Finally, the collective body of work presented here illustrates the value of interdisciplinary collaboration. Virologists, clinicians, entomologists, epidemiologists, data scientists, and public health practitioners each contribute essential perspectives. When these disciplines converge, they generate insights that are greater than the sum of their parts. This Special Issue demonstrates that tackling neglected tropical viral diseases requires not only scientific excellence but also a shared commitment to equity, solidarity, and global health security.

As we look ahead, it is clear that the challenges posed by viral NTDs will continue to evolve. However, the research featured in this Special Issue offers a roadmap for progress, one grounded in innovation, collaboration, and a recognition that no community should be left behind. Continued investment in research, surveillance, and international partnerships will be essential to reduce the burden of these diseases and to build a more resilient and equitable global health landscape.

Institutional Review Board Statement: Not applicable.

Informed Consent Statement: Not applicable.

Data Availability Statement: Not applicable.

Acknowledgments: The Guest Editor thanks all authors and reviewers for their valuable contributions to this Special Issue and acknowledges the editorial office of Tropical Medicine and Infectious Diseases for their support.

Conflicts of Interest: The author declares no conflicts of interest.

References

1. Weaver, S.C.; Reisen, W.K. Present and future arboviral threats. *Antivir. Res.* **2010**, *85*, 328–345. [CrossRef] [PubMed]
2. World Health Organization (WHO). Arboviruses and Human Disease. Available online: https://www.who.int (accessed on 10 January 2026).
3. Wilder-Smith, A.; Gubler, D.J.; Weaver, S.C.; Monath, T.P.; Heymann, D.L.; Scott, T.W. Epidemic arboviral diseases: Priorities for research and public health. *Lancet Infect. Dis.* **2017**, *17*, e101–e106. [CrossRef] [PubMed]
4. Hotez, P.J.; Aksoy, S.; Brindley, P.J.; Kamhawi, S. What constitutes a neglected tropical disease? *PLoS Negl. Trop. Dis.* **2020**, *14*, e0008001. [CrossRef] [PubMed]
5. Abbasi, E. Global expansion of *Aedes* mosquitoes and their role in the transboundary spread of emerging arboviral diseases: A comprehensive review. *IJID One Health* **2025**, *6*, 100058. [CrossRef]
6. Costa-Ribeiro, M.; Krainski, E.; Mello, A.; Carvalho, D.; Luhm, K.; Diaz-Quijano, F.; Raboni, S.; Silva, L.; Buffon, M.; Maluf, E.; et al. Dengue Incidence Following Mass Vaccination: An Interrupted Time Series Study in Paraná, Brazil. *Trop. Med. Infect. Dis.* **2026**, *11*, 11. [CrossRef]

https://doi.org/10.3390/tropicalmed11010029

7. Reigoto, L.; Maciel-de-Freitas, R.; Sikulu-Lord, M.; Garcia, G.; Araujo, G.; Lima, A. Limited Spectroscopy Data and Machine Learning for Detection of Zika Virus Infection in *Aedes aegypti* Mosquitoes. *Trop. Med. Infect. Dis.* **2025**, *10*, 308. [CrossRef] [PubMed]
8. Chandrasena, N.; Ediriweera, D.; Jayakody, D.; Gunathilaka, N.; Premaratna, R. An Overview of Dengue Knowledge, Attitudes, and Practices (KAPs) Among the General Public in Sri Lanka: A Review and Meta-Analysis of Questionnaire-Based Surveys from 2000–2023. *Trop. Med. Infect. Dis.* **2025**, *10*, 189. [CrossRef] [PubMed]
9. To, A.; Kamara, V.; Tekah, D.; Jalloh, M.; Kamara, S.; Wong, T.; Ball, A.; Mayerlen, L.; Ishikawa, K.; Ahn, H.; et al. Baseline Seroprevalence of Arboviruses in Liberia Using a Multiplex IgG Immunoassay. *Trop. Med. Infect. Dis.* **2025**, *10*, 92. [CrossRef] [PubMed]
10. Amaral, J.; Schoen, R.; Weinblatt, M.; Cândido, E. Chikungunya Fever and Rheumatoid Arthritis: A Systematic Review and Meta-Analysis. *Trop. Med. Infect. Dis.* **2025**, *10*, 54. [CrossRef] [PubMed]
11. Melebari, S.; Hafiz, A.; Natto, H.; Elamin, M.; Jalal, N.; Hakim, A.; Rushan, S.; Fallatah, O.; Alzabeedi, K.; Malibari, F.; et al. Estimation and Characterization of Dengue Serotypes in Patients Presenting with Dengue Fever at Makkah Hospitals. *Trop. Med. Infect. Dis.* **2025**, *10*, 27. [CrossRef] [PubMed]
12. He, Y.; Shen, M.; Wang, X.; Yin, A.; Liu, B.; Zhu, J.; Zhang, Z. Suppression of Interferon Response and Antiviral Strategies of Bunyaviruses. *Trop. Med. Infect. Dis.* **2024**, *9*, 205. [CrossRef] [PubMed]
13. Ríos-Bracamontes, E.; Mendoza-Cano, O.; Lugo-Radillo, A.; Ortega-Ramírez, A.; Murillo-Zamora, E. Factors Contributing to In-Hospital Mortality in Dengue: Insights from National Surveillance Data in Mexico (2020–2024). *Trop. Med. Infect. Dis.* **2024**, *9*, 202. [CrossRef] [PubMed]

https://doi.org/10.3390/tropicalmed11010029

Tropical Medicine and Infectious Disease

MDPI

Article

Dengue Incidence Following Mass Vaccination: An Interrupted Time Series Study in Paraná, Brazil

Magda Clara Vieira da Costa-Ribeiro [1,2,*], Elias Teixeira Krainski [3], Angela Maron de Mello [4], Denise Siqueira de Carvalho [2,5], Karin Regina Luhm [2,5], Fredi Alexander Diaz-Quijano [6], Sonia Mara Raboni [5], Lineu Roberto da Silva [5], Marilene da Cruz Magalhães Buffon [2,5], Eliane Mara Cesário Pereira Maluf [5], Gabriel Graef [7], Gustavo Araújo de Almeida [2], Clara Preto [2] and Silvia Emiko Shimakura [8,*]

1 Postgraduate Program in Microbiology, Parasitology and Pathology, Department of Basic Pathology, Federal University of Paraná, Curitiba 80060-000, Brazil
2 Postgraduate Program in Public Health, Federal University of Paraná, Curitiba 80060-240, Brazil; denisecarvalho@ufpr.br (D.S.d.C.); karin.luhm@ufpr.br (K.R.L.); marilenebuffon@ufpr.br (M.d.C.M.B.); almeida.gustavo51@gmail.com (G.A.d.A.); clarampreto@hotmail.com (C.P.)
3 Statistics Program, Computer, Electrical and Mathematical Sciences and Engineering Division, King Abdullah University of Science and Technology, Thuwal 23955-6900, Saudi Arabia; eliaskrainski@gmail.com
4 Health Ministry, Brasília 70058-900, Brazil; angela.maron@gmail.com
5 Department of Public Health, Federal University of Paraná, Curitiba 80060-240, Brazil; sraboni@ufpr.br (S.M.R.); lineu.roberto@ufpr.br (L.R.d.S.); eliane.cesario@ufpr.br (E.M.C.P.M.)
6 Laboratory of Causal Inference in Epidemiology—LINCE-USP, Department of Epidemiology, School of Public Health, University of São Paulo, São Paulo 01246-904, Brazil; frediazq@usp.br
7 Foundation of the Federal University of Paraná (FUNPAR), Curitiba 80010-200, Brazil; gabriel_graeff@hotmail.com
8 Department of Statistics, Federal University of Paraná, Curitiba 81531-890, Brazil
* Correspondence: magdaribeiro@ufpr.br (M.C.V.d.C.-R.); silvia.shimakura@ufpr.br (S.E.S.)

Abstract

In southern Brazil, dengue transmission in the state of Paraná has shown a significant increase in the number of cases since the first recorded occurrence in 1995, with more frequent outbreaks in the west, northwest, and north of the state. We evaluated the impact of a campaign of dengue vaccination administered to a fraction of the population in 30 municipalities in the state by conducting a 15-year interrupted time-series ecological study using data obtained from an official Brazilian data register. We modeled dengue incidence using Poisson regression adjusted by covariates (demographic, climate, and epidemiological factors), allowing for specific temporal variation for each site. A reduction of 18.7% in dengue incidence rate was estimated for a vaccination coverage of 100%. Although there was an increase in the crude dengue incidence rate, considering the three-dose coverage achieved in the municipalities, we estimated an 8.2% relative reduction in the incidence rate. This reduction would increase to 17% with a hypothetical coverage of 90%. The campaign was more effective in small municipalities since they had higher vaccination coverage. These findings underscore the significant impact of the vaccination campaign on reducing dengue incidence trends across the targeted municipalities.

Keywords: dengue; interrupted time-series; vaccine; Dengvaxia®

1. Introduction

In Brazil, dengue has spread since 1986, following an epidemic caused by dengue virus serotype 1 (DENV-1) in the state of Rio de Janeiro [1]. This spread is due to the reintroduction [2] and expansion of the main vector, *Aedes* (*Stegomyia*) *aegypti* (Linnaeus,

1762), as well as factors such as human migration; the occurrence of different serotypes (DENV-1, DENV-2, DENV-3, and DENV-4) and genotypes of the dengue virus [3]; social factors such as population impoverishment; and geographical factors such as climate and environmental changes. Dengue outbreaks follow a cyclical pattern, occurring every three or five years, and the number of cases has been increasing considerably [4]. This indicates that current control measures are not effective enough. The regularity of these cycles, with serotypes alternating between cycles, also suggests the presence of susceptible individuals in the community.

In Paraná state (22°30′58″ to 26°43′00″ S; 48°05′37″ to 54°37′08″ W), which is in southern Brazil, the number of reported dengue cases has been increasing since the first cases were recorded in 1995. Municipalities have reported cases on an annual basis, with the western, northwestern, and northern regions of the state experiencing a higher frequency of dengue circulation. In 2016, all four serotypes of dengue were registered simultaneously. Despite the control measures (cleaning campaigns, insecticide application and educational activities), the state of Paraná has experienced a progressive increase in dengue cases over a period of 21 years [5]. To address this issue, the state opted to vaccinate the population against dengue in 2016 with CYD-TDV (Chimeric Yellow Fever Virus-Dengue Tetravalent Vaccine) Dengvaxia®, the first and only licensed vaccine at the time by the Brazilian National Health Surveillance Agency (Agência Nacional de Vigilância Sanitária—ANVISA) [6]. Thirty priority municipalities with the highest incidence (above 300 per 100,000 inhabitants) recorded in the last five years were selected, and specific age groups for vaccination were targeted. Paraná became second in the world, after the Philippines, in administering the dengue vaccine through the public health system.

Although a previous study has shown that CYD-TDV reduces the risk of dengue among seropositive individuals [7], surveillance data from Paraná revealed a substantial increase in dengue incidence in the years following the mass vaccination campaign. This general rise—likely driven by broader epidemiological dynamics, including the co-circulation of multiple serotypes and the direct and indirect effects of the COVID-19 pandemic—poses challenges to a straightforward assessment of the vaccination impact. Therefore, a key motivation of the present study was the need to estimate the specific contribution of the vaccination campaign on dengue incidence trends by constructing an appropriate counterfactual capable of distinguishing the effect of CYD-TDV from concurrent upward trends in dengue transmission. To address this, we applied a time-series modeling framework incorporating contextual factors and comparisons with unvaccinated municipalities within the same health regions.

2. Materials and Methods

This interrupted time series ecological study was conducted using data obtained from Brazil's Notifiable Diseases Information System (Sistema de Informação de Agravos de Notificação-SINAN) [8–10]. SINAN is a computerized system developed by the Brazilian Ministry of Health for registering mandatory notifiable diseases, including dengue fever [11].

A historical record of dengue fever cases was compiled beginning in 1995. However, the time series analysis was restricted to the period from epidemiological week 1/2008 (1 January 2008) to 36/2022 (5 September 2022). This analysis focused on 10 out of the 22 health regions (Regionais de Saúde; RSs) of the Health Department of Paraná State (SESA/PR): the 1st, 9th, 10th, 12th, 14th, 15th, 17th, 18th, 19th, and 20th RSs. These health regions encompass the 30 municipalities where a portion of the population received the dengue vaccine CYD-TDV (Dengvaxia®) between 16 August 2016, and 18 December 2018.

 https://doi.org/10.3390/tropicalmed11010011

Of the 30 municipalities selected (with >300 DENV cases per 100,000) for the vaccination program, 5 are in the western region, 24 are in the northern region, and 1 is in the eastern region. The vaccine was administered to the population aged between 9 and 44 years in Assaí (18th RS) and Paranaguá (1st RS), and to those aged between 15 and 27 years in the remaining 28 municipalities. Ages were calculated as of August 2016, the start of the vaccination campaign [11] (Figure 1).

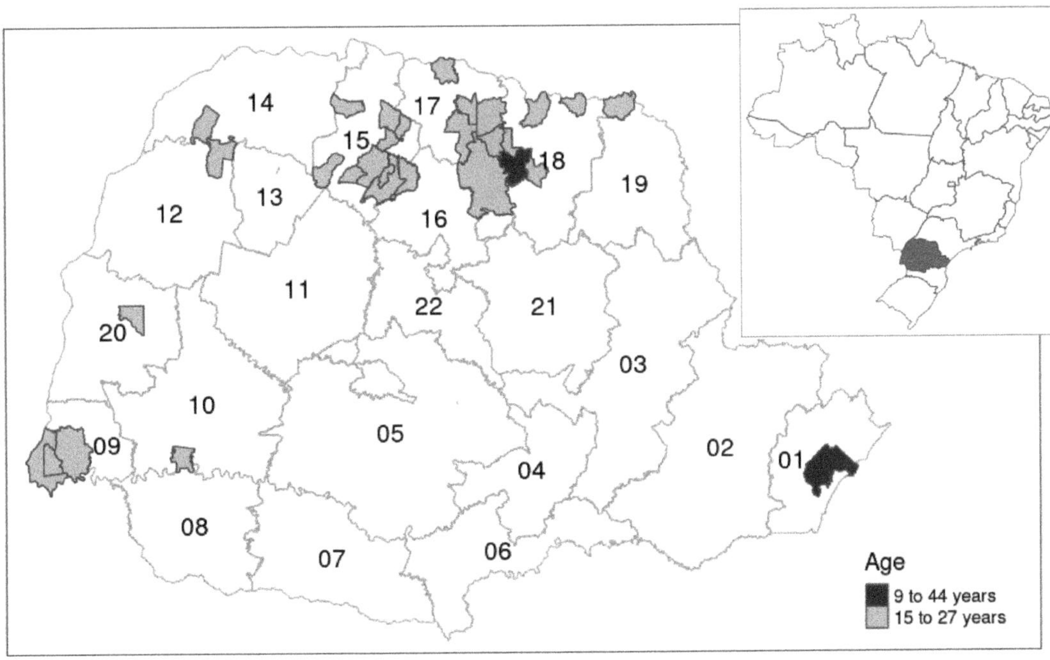

Figure 1. Geographical distribution of vaccinated municipalities in Paraná state, Brazil. Vaccination age range (light gray and black); Health Regions (RS) numbered from 01 to 22 [11].

For each of the 10 RSs, the municipalities that did not receive the vaccine were combined and used as control groups to comparatively assess the impact of the vaccine. The analysis included data from 40 locations, consisting of 30 vaccinated municipalities and 10 groups of unvaccinated municipalities within the 10 targeted RSs. The study analyzed data across three age ranges: (a) cases below the vaccination age range, (b) cases within the vaccination age range, and (c) cases above the vaccination age range. The age ranges were defined according to temporal evolution, with the age range increasing by 1 year each year after 2016. The analysis began when the person received their first vaccine dose (Table 1), and the aim was to track the migration of the age ranges over the course of the study period.

Table 1. Age groups (years) by year, considering age migration, in the 30 municipalities selected for vaccine administration in Paraná state, Brazil.

All Other 28 Municipalities	Assaí and Paranaguá	Year
15 to 27	9 to 44	2016
16 to 28	10 to 45	2017
17 to 29	11 to 46	2018

https://doi.org/10.3390/tropicalmed11010011

Table 1. *Cont.*

All Other 28 Municipalities	Assaí and Paranaguá	Year
18 to 30	12 to 47	2019
19 to 31	13 to 48	2020
20 to 32	14 to 49	2021
21 to 33	15 to 50	2022

2.1. The Reference Population for Calculating the Incidence Rate

The population data for each municipality used in this study were obtained from the Brazilian Institute of Geography and Statistics (Instituto Brasileiro de Geografia e Estatística; IBGE) for the years 2008–2009 and 2011–2021, via the IBGE Automatic Recovery System (Sistema IBGE de Recuperação Automática). The IBGE is a federal government agency responsible for collecting annual population data for all municipalities in the country. The population reference for the year 2010 was based on the census conducted that year and divided by age groups. For the year 2022, a growth rate of 9.94% was applied, with the estimated numbers based on the population of previous years as to the date of this analysis in the 2022 Census Reports that had not yet been released. The resulting data include population numbers for each municipality and year, which are divided into three age groups (Supplementary Material S1).

2.2. Time Series Model

The output of the adopted model is the weekly count of dengue cases in each of the 40 locations, segmented by age group, resulting in 120 weekly time series. To model the relative incidence risk, we used the population data aggregated by age group and year (Supplementary Material S1).

The statistical model was adjusted for the time series, y_{ikt}, with $i = 1, \ldots, 40$, indicating the location i; $k = 1, 2, 3$ representing the age range and $t = 1, ..., 766$, indicating week t, where $t = 1$ is the first epidemiological week of 2008 and $t = 766$ is the 36th epidemiological week of 2022.

The expected number of cases, assuming that the population in location i, age group k, and epidemiological week t has a similar rate to the overall gross rate of the 10 RSs, is calculated as

$$E_{ikt} = m_0 \times P_{ika}/n_a, \quad (1)$$

where P_{ika} is the population in location i, age group k, and year a, which is repeated for every epidemiological week t within year a; n_a is the number of epidemiological weeks in year a; and m_0 is the annual gross rate (baseline rate) obtained from the absolute incidence in the 10 RSs over the entire period, obtained by

$$m_0 = \frac{\sum_{i=1}^{40} \sum_{a=1}^{15} \sum_{k=1}^{3} y_{ika}}{\sum_{i=1}^{40} \sum_{a=1}^{15} \sum_{k=1}^{3} P_{ika}}, \quad (2)$$

where y_{ika} is the number of dengue cases in location i, age group k, and year a, for $k = 1, 2, 3$; $a = 1, ..., 15$ (with $a = 1$ being the year 2008) and $i = 1, ..., 40$.

A Poisson distribution was assumed for $\mathrm{y_{ikt}}$

$$y_{ikt} \sim \text{Poisson}(E_{ikt} \times \lambda_{ikt}),$$

where λ_{ikt} is the hazard ratio of location i, age group k relative to the baseline rate at week t.

 https://doi.org/10.3390/tropicalmed11010011

The factors adjusted in the model for the hazard ratio λ_{itk} were exposure (the weekly coverage of the full course of three doses of vaccination in each municipality); control variables (the circulating serotype in each RS per year); age group (with the vaccinated group as the reference group); a specific temporal variation for each location; and a climate variable calculated from an estimated time series of daily minimum temperature in each location. The climate variable used was the proportion of time in the week when the minimum temperature was above 21 °C, lagged by week (from 0 to 15 weeks) [12–19] (Supplementary Material S2).

2.3. Vaccination Coverage

To evaluate whether the vaccination coverage with three doses is associated with the number of cases, an index was calculated that varies over time; the accumulated proportion of the target population vaccinated with three doses (VC), which reflects the weekly vaccination coverage of three doses for each municipality. Coverage is zero before the start of vaccination and reaches the maximum level (three doses) of that municipality at the end of the vaccination period, December 2018.

2.4. Vaccination Effectiveness

After adjusting the model, we used Formula (3) to quantify the effectiveness of the vaccine campaign in a municipality with a VC × 100% coverage of three doses of the vaccine:

$$\text{effectiveness} = (1 - \exp(\beta \times \text{VC})) \times 100\% \tag{3}$$

where β represents the estimated effect of vaccine coverage, and VC ($0 \leq \text{VC} \leq 1$) is the coverage rate of three vaccine doses.

2.5. Predictions from Two Scenarios

To compare the effectiveness of the vaccine, the model was used to predict the expected number of cases in two hypothetical scenarios for the target population of the vaccine in the 30 municipalities:

Scenario 1: No vaccine dose was applied (0% coverage).

Scenario 2: High percentage of the population in the vaccine age group received three doses (90% coverage).

To predict the number of cases under these scenarios, we used 3000 independent samples (Monte Carlo) from the approximate joint distribution of all model parameters. These scenarios were evaluated from 2 January 2019 (15 days after the end of the vaccination program), to 5 September 2022 (end of the study).

This procedure allows for hypothetical scenarios to be drawn and predicts the expected vaccination effects on the number of dengue cases under varying vaccination coverage conditions, assuming that other conditions, such as circulating serotypes and weather conditions, remain as observed.

In Scenario 1, we determine the reduction in the number of cases attributed to the vaccination campaign by subtracting the observed number of cases from the number of cases predicted by the model under a 0% coverage assumption. This considers each location's final three-dose coverage rate. To calculate the reduction in cases in Scenario 2, we compare the predicted number of cases under a 90% coverage scenario (which simulates a successful vaccination campaign) to the predicted number of cases under a no vaccination scenario. The predicted number of cases also includes 95% credible intervals to account for the observed coverage and predicted cases under both scenarios.

The R package INLA [18], version 22.04.16, was used considering the central composite design (CCD) strategy for the experimental design to integrate with respect to the three

https://doi.org/10.3390/tropicalmed11010011

hyperparameters of the model. All the statistical analyses were performed via the R statistical analysis system [20].

3. Results

3.1. Dengue Incidence and Serotypes

Paraná state, initially characterized by dengue cases reported in 16 municipalities in 1995, has since expanded to 347 additional municipalities reporting cases as of 2022, resulting in a total of 363 affected municipalities. The vaccinated municipalities were those with consistently high incidence rates, driving the state's overall pattern (Figure 2).

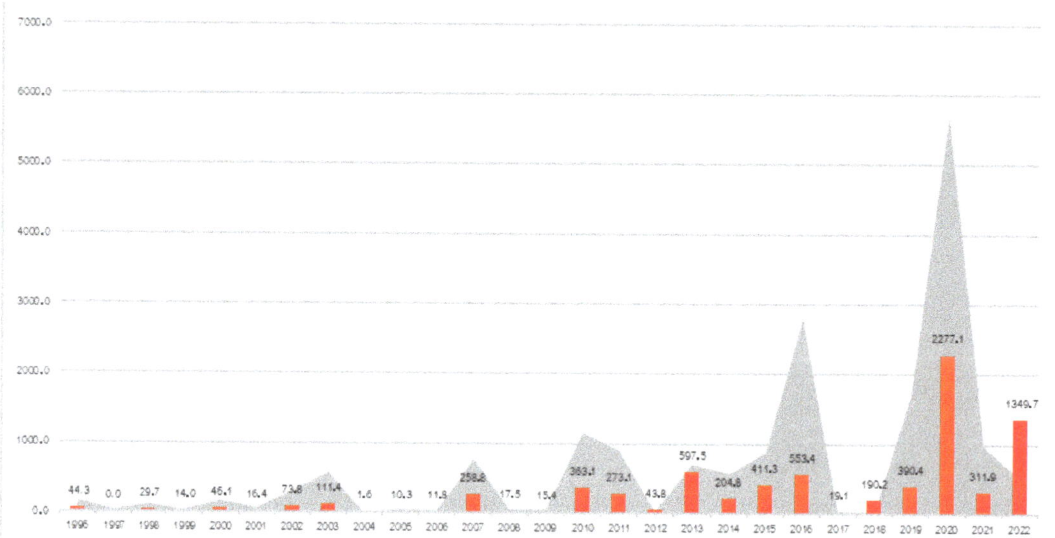

Figure 2. Annual dengue incidence rates per 100,000 inhabitants in 30 municipalities of Paraná state from 1995 to 2022. Municipalities incidence rate (gray); Paraná incidence rate (red).

During the analyzed period, 1,379,141 dengue cases were reported in Paraná, of which 609,632 were of autochthonous origin. After excluding 2161 notifications classified as "discarded" and 482 as "not assessed", 606,989 probable autochthonous cases were observed in the state, hereafter referred to as "cases" (Table 2).

Table 2. Dengue notifications according to SINAN, Paraná state, from 1 January 2008 to 5 September 2022.

Final Classification	Autochthonous Origin				Total	
	Indefinite	N.A.	No	Yes	*N*	%
Dengue	2008	33,666	17,874	595,212	648,760	47.0
Dengue with warning signs	35	408	199	7458	8100	0.6
Severe dengue	12	40	48	1396	1496	0.1
Inconclusive	395	60,744	492	2923	64,554	4.7
Probable cases	2450	94,858	18,613	606,989	722,910	52.4
Discarded	54	640,163	7113	2161	649,491	47.1
N.A.	6	6211	41	482	6740	0.5
Total	2510	741,232	25,767	609,632	1,379,141	100.0

N.A.: Not Assessed.

The 30 municipalities selected for vaccination had 271,114 cases during the specified period. The other 172 municipalities in the same 10 RSs where the vaccination campaign

 https://doi.org/10.3390/tropicalmed11010011

took place that did not participate in the campaign reported 293,940 cases. The remaining municipalities in Paraná had 41,935 cases that were excluded from the analysis, resulting in a total of 565,054 cases (Table 2). Among the municipalities scheduled to receive the vaccine, Londrina had the highest proportion of cases, accounting for 25.1% of the total, followed by Foz do Iguaçu with 23.4% and Maringá with 12.0%, making up a total of 60.5% of the cases. For the unvaccinated municipalities, the cases were more evenly distributed across the 10 RSs, with the highest percentages in the 14th RS (17.8%), the 20th RS (15.4%), the 10th RS (15.2%), the 15th RS (11.7%), and the 12th RS (11.4%) of the cases, accounting for 71.5% of the cases (Table 3).

Table 3. Frequency of dengue cases in municipalities located in the 10 health regions of Paraná state, Brazil, participants and non-participants of the dengue vaccination campaign from 1 January 2008 to 5 September 2022.

<table>
<tr><th>Vaccinated Municipalities</th><th>N</th><th>%</th><th>Health Region (Unvaccinated Municipalities)</th><th>N</th><th>%</th></tr>
<tr><td>Paranaguá</td><td>18,577</td><td>6.9</td><td>RS 01 (6)</td><td>4326</td><td>1.5</td></tr>
<tr><td>Foz do Iguaçu</td><td>63,440</td><td>23.4</td><td rowspan="3">RS 09 (6)</td><td rowspan="3">16,701</td><td rowspan="3">5.7</td></tr>
<tr><td>SM Iguaçu</td><td>2964</td><td>1.1</td></tr>
<tr><td>ST Itaipu</td><td>4321</td><td>1.6</td></tr>
<tr><td>Boa Vista da Aparecida</td><td>343</td><td>0.1</td><td>RS 10 (24)</td><td>44,603</td><td>15.2</td></tr>
<tr><td>Tapira</td><td>1205</td><td>0.4</td><td>RS 12 (20)</td><td>33,417</td><td>11.4</td></tr>
<tr><td>Cruzeiro do Sul</td><td>1009</td><td>0.4</td><td rowspan="2">RS 14 (26)</td><td rowspan="2">52,466</td><td rowspan="2">17.8</td></tr>
<tr><td>Santa Isabel do Ivaí</td><td>3386</td><td>1.2</td></tr>
<tr><td>Iguaraçu</td><td>613</td><td>0.2</td><td rowspan="9">RS 15 (21)</td><td rowspan="9">34,361</td><td rowspan="9">11.7</td></tr>
<tr><td>Munhoz Melo</td><td>550</td><td>0.2</td></tr>
<tr><td>Mandaguari</td><td>2520</td><td>0.9</td></tr>
<tr><td>Marialva</td><td>3171</td><td>1.2</td></tr>
<tr><td>Maringá</td><td>32,624</td><td>12.0</td></tr>
<tr><td>Paiçandu</td><td>4086</td><td>1.5</td></tr>
<tr><td>Santa Fé</td><td>2299</td><td>0.8</td></tr>
<tr><td>Sarandi</td><td>15,830</td><td>5.8</td></tr>
<tr><td>SJ Ivaí</td><td>1111</td><td>0.4</td></tr>
<tr><td>Assaí</td><td>4205</td><td>1.6</td><td rowspan="8">RS 17 (13)</td><td rowspan="8">28,034</td><td rowspan="8">9.5</td></tr>
<tr><td>Bela Vista do Paraíso</td><td>2712</td><td>1.0</td></tr>
<tr><td>Cambé</td><td>12,575</td><td>4.6</td></tr>
<tr><td>Ibiporã</td><td>6500</td><td>2.4</td></tr>
<tr><td>Jataizinho</td><td>5448</td><td>2.0</td></tr>
<tr><td>Londrina</td><td>68,036</td><td>25.1</td></tr>
<tr><td>Porecatu</td><td>4020</td><td>1.5</td></tr>
<tr><td>Sertanópolis</td><td>4346</td><td>1.6</td></tr>
<tr><td>Itambaracá</td><td>649</td><td>0.2</td><td rowspan="3">RS 18 (18)</td><td rowspan="3">21,836</td><td rowspan="3">7.4</td></tr>
<tr><td>Leópolis</td><td>295</td><td>0.1</td></tr>
<tr><td>SS Amoreira</td><td>1238</td><td>0.5</td></tr>
<tr><td>Cambará</td><td>2044</td><td>0.8</td><td>RS 19 (21)</td><td>13,018</td><td>4.4</td></tr>
<tr><td>Maripá</td><td>997</td><td>0.4</td><td>RS 20 (17)</td><td>45,178</td><td>15.4</td></tr>
<tr><td>Total</td><td>271,114</td><td>100</td><td>Total</td><td>293,940</td><td>100.0</td></tr>
</table>

Between 2008 and 2022, the DENV-3 serotype was the least frequently detected (in three years), followed by DENV-4 (in 9 years) and DENV-2 (in 11 years) (Figure 3). DENV-1 was the most prevalent virus in this period and presented high incidence rates, except in 2020, when more than 80% of the identified virus was DENV-2 [5].

https://doi.org/10.3390/tropicalmed11010011

The group of municipalities selected for vaccination had the highest incidence rate of dengue in 2016 among the age groups eligible for vaccination. From 2019 to 2021, the rates were even higher for all age groups in the municipalities participating in vaccination (Participant) than in the unvaccinated group (Non-participant). However, in 2022, the situation was reversed, with higher dengue rates in the unvaccinated group across all age groups (Figure 4).

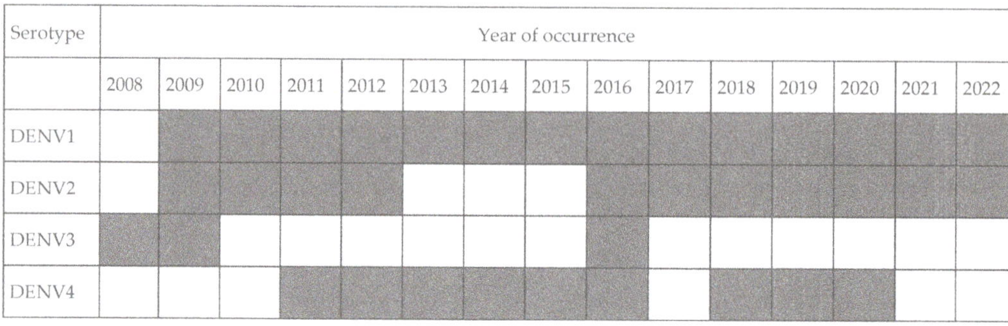

Figure 3. Serotypes identified by year from 2008 to 2022, Paraná state, Brazil. Adapted from [5].

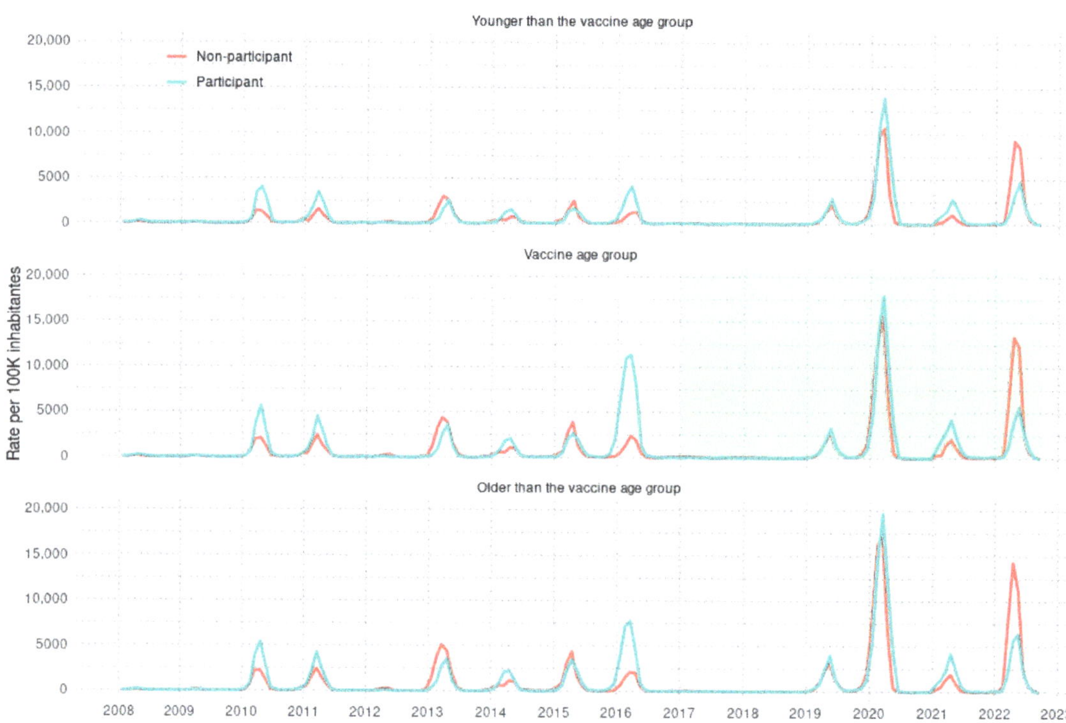

Figure 4. Monthly dengue incidence rates (per 100,000 inhabitants) by age groups in municipalities in Paraná state, participating in vaccination versus municipalities not participating in vaccination from 2008 to 2022. The green area in the vaccine age group panel shows the period of time six months after the beginning of the vaccination.

The aggregated incidence rates for the pre-vaccine (2008–2015) and post-vaccine (2019–2022) periods by age group (vaccine age range, below and above the vaccine age

https://doi.org/10.3390/tropicalmed11010011

range), as well as the RRs, are presented in Table 4. The incidence rates during the post-vaccine period were higher than those during the pre-vaccine period, both within and outside the vaccine age range. However, the magnitude of the RR was lower in municipalities where vaccination was conducted in each age group. For example, in the targeted age range, the RR for the post-vaccine period compared with the pre-vaccine period was 2.4 in vaccinated municipalities, whereas it was 4.4 in unvaccinated municipalities.

Table 4. Dengue incidence rates per 100,000 inhabitants and rate ratios, according to vaccination participation group and age group, in the 10 health regions of Paraná state, Brazil, during the pre-vaccination (2008–2015) and post-vaccination (2019–2022) periods.

Period	Group	Within the Eligible Age Range for Vaccination	Age Group Below the Eligible Age Range for Vaccination	Above the Eligible Age Range for Vaccination
Pre-vaccination period	Participant	17	9.4	14
	Non-participant	9.4	6.3	10
Post-vaccination period	Participant	40.3	30.6	43.2
	Non-participant	41.7	28.7	44.6
RR * (Post/Pre)	Participant	2.4	3.3	3.1
	Non-participant	4.4	4.6	4.5

*** Rate Ratio**

Weekly time series of incidence rates for the three age ranges were higher in the municipalities of Tapira (12th RS), São Jorge do Ivaí (15th RS), Porecatu (17th RS), São Sebastião da Amoreira (18th RS), Cambará (19th RS), and Maripá (20th RS) in 2022 than in unvaccinated municipalities in the same RS. In 2020, in Foz do Iguaçu (9th RS), dengue caused by serotype DENV-2 affected all age groups, including vaccinated individuals, with incidence rates much higher than 300 per 100,000 inhabitants. High rates also occurred in the other two municipalities that received the vaccine; however, in the vaccinated group, they were slightly lower than in the rest of the region. However, in 2022, these municipalities showed higher incidence rates compared to Foz do Iguaçu, where rates were lower, and the predominant virus was DENV-1.

3.2. Vaccine Coverage

The weekly time series of the number of third doses of the dengue vaccine shows three decreasing peaks over time (Figure 5A). The largest peak occurred in the second half of 2017, the intermediate peak at the beginning of 2018, and the smallest at the end of 2018, which marked the finish of the vaccination campaign. The time series of the weekly vaccination coverage for three doses per participating municipality in the vaccination campaign shows significant variability in vaccination coverage (Figure 5B).

https://doi.org/10.3390/tropicalmed11010011

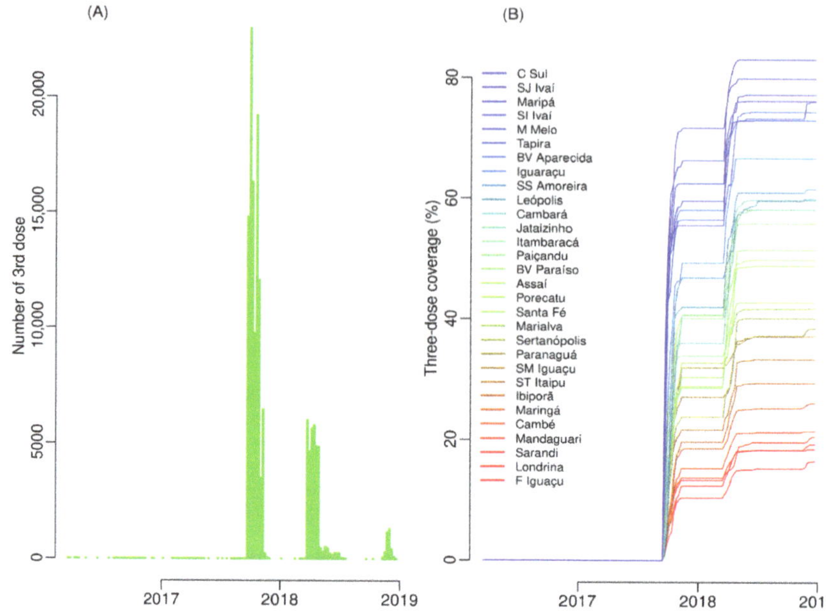

Figure 5. Evolution of the proportion of people vaccinated against dengue, with three doses over time, in 30 municipalities of Paraná state from 2016 to 2018, Brazil. (**A**) Weekly number of people vaccinated with three doses; (**B**) Weekly coverage of three vaccine doses.

3.3. Time Series Analysis

The climate variable was adjusted in the model by considering different time lags, and the lags between 9 and 12 weeks showed the best fit. They were combined into a common factor (the proportion of time during the period of 9–12 weeks before the date of the cases when the minimum hourly temperature exceeded 21 °C) and used in the final model [12–19] (Supplementary Material S2).

The estimated effect of vaccination coverage −0.207 (95% CI = [−0.252; −0.161]) was significantly less than zero, resulting in a reduction in the hazard ratio of dengue cases (HR = 0.813; 95% CI = [0.777; 0.851]).

The effectiveness of the vaccine campaign for a (vaccination coverage of 100%) was estimated from this result as 18.7% (95%CI = [14.9%; 22.3%]) [21–23] (Supplementary Material S3). This percentage reduction in cases is expected in a hypothetical scenario where a municipality has 100% coverage of the third vaccine dose. However, none of the study locations achieved vaccination coverage of 100%. The municipality with the highest vaccination coverage of three doses was Cruzeiro do Sul, with 83.0%, and in this case, the campaign's effectiveness was estimated to be 15.8%. In contrast, the municipality with the lowest vaccination coverage was Foz do Iguaçu, with only 16.4% of its population vaccinated, resulting in an estimated effectiveness of $(1 - exp(-0.207 \times 0.164)) \cdot 100\% = 3.3\%$.

The estimated specific temporal variation for each location after adjusting for all the observed factors, along with their 95% credible intervals estimated under the model, are represented in Figure 6. Different patterns are observed in the series, both in terms of their profiles and error margins. However, neighboring municipalities, such as Maringá and Sarandi and Londrina and Cambé, tended to exhibit similar patterns of cyclical variation in dengue. Interestingly, Paranaguá's specific temporal variation was low until 2016 and the highest in 2016 compared with the other locations. In fact, dengue was introduced in Paranaguá in 2016, and it had the highest observed rate.

 https://doi.org/10.3390/tropicalmed11010011

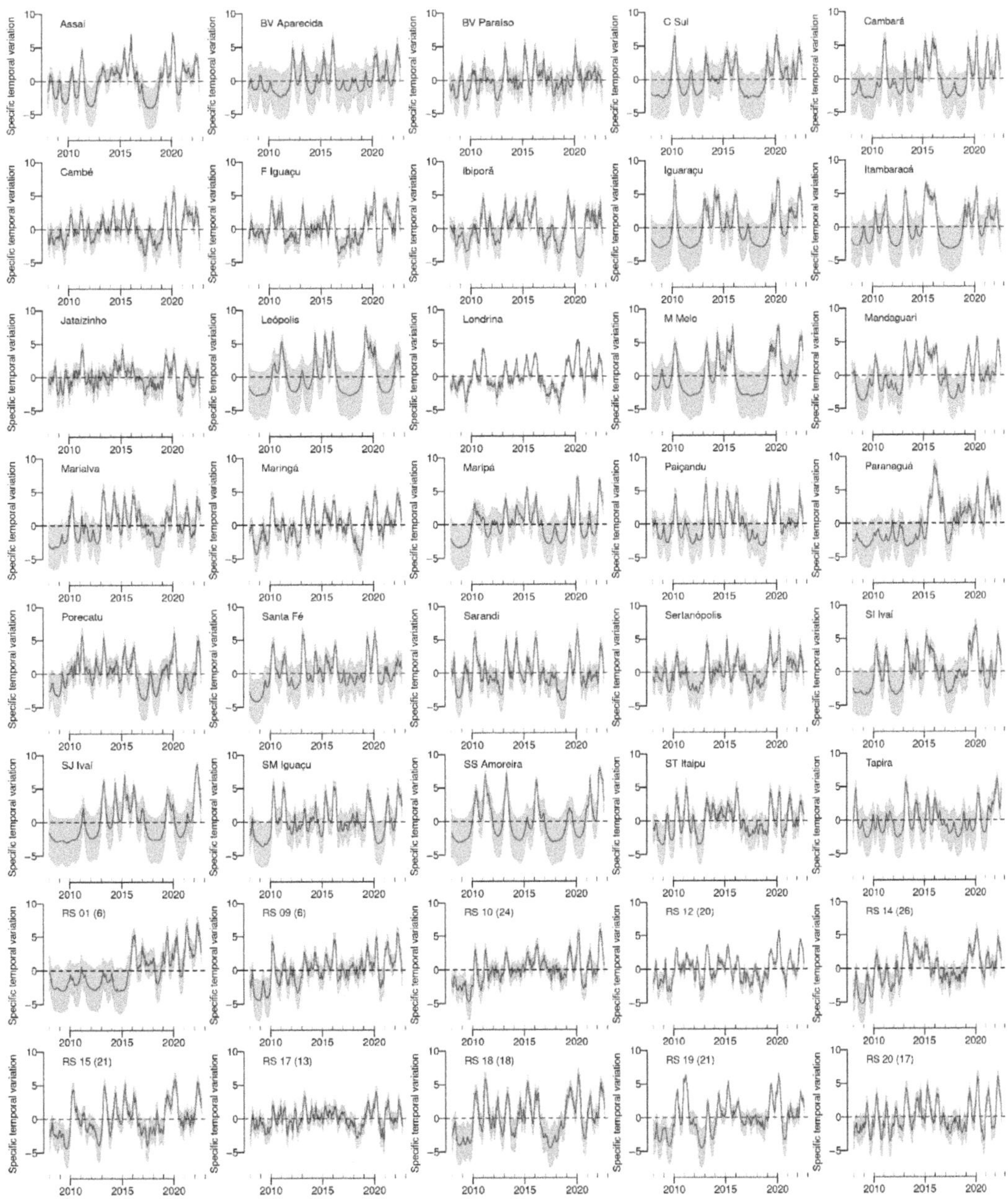

Figure 6. Estimated specific temporal variation for each location (black line) and 95% credible intervals (grey color) in Paraná state, Brazil.

The findings from the first scenario suggest that there was an 8.2% decrease in the number of dengue cases due to the vaccination campaign. This means that there were 3411 fewer cases than what the model had predicted in the absence of the vaccination. For a three-dose vaccination coverage reaching 90% (Scenario 2), the expected overall reduction in dengue cases across all 30 municipalities was 17.0%, corresponding to 7090 fewer cases (Supplementary Material S4).

https://doi.org/10.3390/tropicalmed11010011

4. Discussion

Between 2008 and 2015, the western, northwestern, and northern regions of the state of Paraná recorded the highest number of dengue cases. It was only in 2016, in the eastern region, specifically in the city of Paranaguá, that the first significant epidemic of DENV-1 occurred on the state coast [24]. The history of DENV infection varied among the 30 municipalities selected for vaccination. Londrina had the highest number of cases (68,036), followed by Foz do Iguaçu (63,440) and Maringá (32,624), whereas Munhoz de Melo (550), Boa Vista da Aparecida (343), and Leópolis (295) had the lowest number of cases. However, the highest incidence until 2016 was observed in small municipalities.

In a previous vaccine effectiveness study using individual-level data, we demonstrated that CYD-TDV (Dengvaxia®) was associated with a 21.3% reduction in the risk of dengue, with the effect being modified by a history of dengue [7]. In this new study, we documented the significant impact of the vaccination campaign on the incidence rate trend. As expected, the overall population impact of the campaign was statistically significant, dependent on vaccine coverage, and independent of contextual factors. The proposed model included covariates, such as the circulating serotypes, population density, temperature, and age within the recommended vaccination range.

Our findings indicate that larger municipalities act as modulators of seasonal DENV transmission patterns at the regional level, whereas smaller municipalities (<10,000 inhabitants) show seasonal patterns that are largely determined by the epidemiological context of their surrounding regions.

Temperature is one of the key factors affecting survival, longevity, vector capacity, and other aspects of the life cycle of *Ae. aegypti* [25]. In this study, temperature was identified as a risk factor (HR = 3.49 95% CI = [2.73; 4.49]) for the dengue virus. In a temporal and spatial analysis, the high incidence rates of dengue and the heterogeneous spatial distribution in the state of Paraná were attributed to sociodemographic factors and environmental determinants [26].

For the model, the DENV-1 serotype was the only one that presented a significant risk factor (HR = 3.49 95% CI = [2.73; 4.49]) for the occurrence of dengue epidemics. Proportionally, DENV-1 was the serotype that was present in the state for the longest period. One probable explanation for this is the introduction of new variants and the genetic diversity of DENV-1 [27]. The V genotype (American/African), which is grouped in the clade of lineages I, II, and III, was detected for this serotype in Brazil [28]. The lowest risk was attributed to DENV-3, followed by DENV-2 and DENV-4. DENV-2 was the first serotype to circulate in the southern region of the country, and it was introduced in the state of Paraná in 1995. DENV-1 was introduced in Santa Catarina in 1999, DENV-3 in Paraná in 2000, and DENV-4 in Rio Grande do Sul in 2011 [29].

The highest degree of vaccination coverage was observed in municipalities with fewer than 10,000 inhabitants, as previously reported [11]. Among these municipalities, Cruzeiro do Sul had the highest coverage rate at 83.0%, resulting in a higher estimated effectiveness rate of 15.8% (95% CI = [12.5%; 18.9%]). Conversely, Foz do Iguaçu had the lowest coverage rate at 16.4%, resulting in a lower effectiveness rate of 3.3% (95% CI = [2.6%; 4.0%]). The overall effectiveness rate across all 30 municipalities was 18.7% (95% CI = [14.9%; 22.3%]). Despite the high variability in vaccination coverage, with 33% of municipalities having a coverage rate of 40% or less and low vaccine effectiveness, the two scenario predictions suggest an overall reduction of 8.2% in dengue cases when three vaccine doses are considered. The approach used includes a vaccination coverage indicator that varies over time, ranging from 0% coverage before the start of vaccination to the achieved coverage level in each municipality, which could reach 95% of the target population.

https://doi.org/10.3390/tropicalmed11010011

In the analysis of the incidence rates (unadjusted), there was a generalized increase in dengue cases after the vaccination period. However, in the municipalities where the vaccine was implemented, the rate ratio in the vaccinated age group was the lowest (RR = 2.4), suggesting a possible vaccine effect. According to the statistical model, individuals below and above the vaccinated age group presented a lower risk for dengue infections. However, Paranaguá, one of the municipalities that targeted the age group of 9–45 years, experienced the first dengue epidemic between 2014 and 2016 [24]. The co-circulation of multiple dengue serotypes reduces adults' susceptibility due to acquired immunity from the disease [30]. In Paraná, the highest incidence rate was reported in the population aged between 20 and 59 years, with a significant difference in the incidence rate between age groups: ≤10 years ($p < 0.01$), ≥60 years ($p < 0.05$), and 11–19 years ($p < 0.05$) [26]. Furthermore, a global analysis revealed that individuals under 5 years of age, the age group previously responsible for most deaths and years of life lost due to dengue in 1990, were replaced by those between 15 and 49 years of age in 2019 [31].

Dengue epidemics are complex and multifactorial [26,32]. Brazil is experiencing a hyperendemic scenario, with the co-circulation of all four serotypes of DENV and an increasing occurrence of severe and fatal cases, as well as the co-circulation of other arboviruses, such as Zika, yellow fever, and Chikungunya [31].

The susceptibility of the human population to circulating serotypes and their genotypes, as well as the mosquito infestation index, are factors related to the number of dengue cases [33]. Moreover, climatic, environmental, social, and demographic factors, as well as vector control measures, also play a significant role in its incidence.

Several limiting factors made it difficult to adjust the model during the study. For example, it was challenging to obtain a representative sample of the circulating serotype and its genotypes. In our previous study using individual data from confirmed cases, we reported that the vaccine effectively reduced the risk for certain serotypes (DENV-1 and DENV-4) but had no such effect on DENV-2. In fact, in patients without prior dengue infection, the vaccine increased the risk of DENV-2. Thus, the circulating serotype is a key factor in determining the impact of a vaccine. In the present study, which focused on probable cases (most of which lacked serotype data), we were unable to disaggregate cases by serotype. Nevertheless, the significant reduction in probable cases indicates that the benefits of vaccination outweigh any adverse effects. The heterogeneity of the efficacy of this vaccine has already been documented in clinical trials [34]. Thus, it is well accepted that a seronegative status implies a lack of benefit. Therefore, the vaccine would be indicated only for seropositive individuals. Since the campaign was carried out before this knowledge was available, there would be concern about the population impact of the mass vaccination program. In this sense, our study contributes to assessing the impact from the perspective of its association with the incidence rate of probable cases. These results complement previously published estimates that focused on confirmed cases [7,35].

Additionally, historical data on dengue in the target municipalities and data on the infestation of *Ae. aegypti* were unavailable. Another issue was the limited number of meteorological stations in the state.

It is important to acknowledge that dengue incidence increased markedly across the state during the post-vaccination period, reflecting the influence of factors that were unrelated to the intervention. The COVID-19 pandemic, for example, may have affected viral circulation patterns, health-seeking behavior, reporting practices, and vector control activities, potentially amplifying dengue transmission. Moreover, the predominance of particular serotypes, especially DENV-2 during certain years, may have attenuated the population-level impact of the vaccine, given known differences in vaccine performance by serostatus and serotype.

https://doi.org/10.3390/tropicalmed11010011

Despite these strong external pressures, our modeling results indicate that the increase in dengue incidence was smaller than expected in municipalities that implemented vaccination when compared with the estimated counterfactual scenario. In other words, although the crude trends show an overall rise, the vaccination campaign appears to have mitigated part of this increase. This finding aligns with previous evidence of CYD-TDV's individual-level effectiveness and reinforces that the campaign's impact should be interpreted as a relative reduction in expected incidence, rather than as prevention of outbreaks under the highly unfavorable epidemiological conditions of recent years.

These observations underscore the importance of accounting for secular trends, serotype dynamics, and concurrent public health disruptions when evaluating population-level vaccine impact. Relying solely on crude pre-post comparisons would risk underestimating the benefits of the campaign, whereas the counterfactual modeling framework allows a more accurate estimation of its marginal effect.

5. Conclusions

An analysis of the unadjusted incidence rates revealed a general increase in dengue occurrence during the post-vaccination period across the state. In this context of rising transmission, the time-series model indicated that municipalities implementing the vaccination campaign experienced a lower-than-expected increase in dengue incidence when compared with the counterfactual scenario. After adjusting for serotype circulation, climatic conditions, age structure, and location-specific temporal patterns, vaccination coverage was associated with a significant reduction in the risk of dengue. According to model-based predictions, the campaign prevented an estimated 8.2% of cases under the coverage levels achieved, and this reduction could have reached 17% with higher vaccination coverage. These findings suggest that, despite the strong upward secular trends in recent years, the mass vaccination campaign contributed to mitigating the expected burden of dengue in the targeted municipalities.

Supplementary Materials: The following supporting information can be downloaded at: https://www.mdpi.com/article/10.3390/tropicalmed11010011/s1, Material S1: Estimated populations for three age groups (below vaccination range, within vaccination range, above vaccination range) by municipality and year; Material S2: Methodology for creating the climate variable; Material S3: Estimates and 95% credibility intervals of posterior of model effects and observed versus predicted series; Material S4: Time series with results of prediction scenarios.

Author Contributions: Conceptualization, S.E.S., M.C.V.d.C.-R., A.M.d.M. and E.T.K.; methodology, S.E.S., M.C.V.d.C.-R., A.M.d.M. and E.T.K.; software, E.T.K.; validation, E.T.K. and S.E.S.; formal analysis, E.T.K., S.E.S., M.C.V.d.C.-R. and A.M.d.M.; investigation, M.C.V.d.C.-R., E.T.K., A.M.d.M., D.S.d.C., K.R.L., F.A.D.-Q., S.M.R., L.R.d.S., M.d.C.M.B., E.M.C.P.M., G.G., G.A.d.A., C.P. and S.E.S.; resources, D.S.d.C. and K.R.L.; data curation, S.E.S. and E.T.K.; writing—original draft preparation, M.C.V.d.C.-R., A.M.d.M. and S.E.S.; writing—review and editing, M.C.V.d.C.-R., A.M.d.M., S.E.S., F.A.D.-Q. and S.M.R.; visualization, M.C.V.d.C.-R., E.T.K., A.M.d.M., D.S.d.C., K.R.L., F.A.D.-Q., S.M.R., L.R.d.S., M.d.C.M.B., E.M.C.P.M., G.G., G.A.d.A., C.P. and S.E.S.; supervision, S.E.S.; project administration, D.S.d.C. and K.R.L.; funding acquisition, D.S.d.C. and K.R.L. All authors have read and agreed to the published version of the manuscript.

Funding: This work was supported by Sanofi Pasteur. The funder of this collaborative study participated in discussing the study's findings and reviewing the manuscript. The authors analyzed and interpreted the data and submitted the manuscript for publication. Registered in the institution's Integrated Agreement Management System under Process number 23075.168655/2017-62.

Institutional Review Board Statement: This study was approved by the Research Ethics Committee of the Federal University of Paraná (No. 2.308.662) in 30 November 2016.

https://doi.org/10.3390/tropicalmed11010011

Informed Consent Statement: This study did not require an informed consent statement because it relied exclusively on secondary data. This data consists of official and publicly available information obtained in aggregated form (as counts) within the defined geographic regions of the study.

Data Availability Statement: The datasets used and/or analyzed during the current study are available from the corresponding author upon reasonable request.

Acknowledgments: We would like to thank the Paraná's State Health Department Work Group, specially Júlia Valéria Ferreira Cordellini, João Luís Gallego Crivellaro and Raul Júnior Belly for granting access to the dengue nominal vaccine registry. We are grateful to all contributors and reviewers who dedicated their valuable time and expertise to developing this Special Issue.

Conflicts of Interest: The authors declare no conflicts of interest. The funders had no role in the study's design; in the collection, analyses, or interpretation of data; in the writing of the manuscript; or in the decision to publish the results.

Abbreviations

The following abbreviations are used in this manuscript:

DENV-1	Dengue Virus serotype 1
DENV-2	Dengue Virus serotype 2
DENV-3	Dengue Virus serotype 3
DENV-4	Dengue Virus serotype 4
CYD-TDV	Chimeric Yellow Fever Virus-Dengue Tetravalent Vaccine
ANVISA	Agência Nacional de Vigilância Sanitária
SINAN	Sistema de Informação de Agravos de Notificação
RS	Regional de Saúde
SESA	Secretaria de Estado da Saúde
PR	Paraná
IBGE	Instituto Brasileiro de Geografia e Estatística
VC	Vaccination Coverage
CCD	Central Composite Design
RR	Rate Ratio
CI	Confidence Interval/Credible Interval
HR	Hazard Ratio

References

1. Schatzmayr, H.G.; Nogueira, R.M.R.; da Rosa, A.P.A.T. An outbreak of dengue virus at Rio de Janeiro-1986. *Mem. Inst. Oswaldo Cruz* **1986**, *81*, 245–246. [CrossRef] [PubMed]
2. Braga, I.A.; Valle, D. *Aedes aegypti*: Inseticidas, mecanismos de ação e resistência. *Epidemiol. Serv. Saúde* **2007**, *16*, 179–293. [CrossRef]
3. de Jesus, J.G.; Dutra, K.R.; Sales, F.C.d.S.; Claro, I.M.; Terzian, A.C.; Candido, D.d.S.; Hill, S.C.; Thézé, J.; Torres, C.; D'aGostini, T.L.; et al. Genomic detection of a virus lineage replacement event of dengue virus serotype 2 in Brazil, 2019. *Mem. Do Inst. Oswaldo Cruz* **2020**, *115*, e190423. [CrossRef] [PubMed]
4. PAHO. As Dengue Cases Increase Globally, Vector Control, Community Engagement Key to Prevent Spread of the Disease. 2023. Available online: https://www.paho.org/en/news/3-8-2023-dengue-cases-increase-globally-vector-control-community-engagement-key-prevent-spread (accessed on 5 August 2024).
5. Boletim Epidemiológico. Informe Epidemiológico 47/2023-2024. 2024. Available online: https://seer.uftm.edu.br/revistaeletronica/index.php/revistatriangulo/article/download/7868/8408/48869 (accessed on 10 December 2025).
6. Conass. Paraná Inicia Campanha Inédita de Vacinação Contra a Dengue. 2016. Available online: https://www.conass.org.br/6873-2/ (accessed on 5 August 2024).
7. Diaz-Quijano, F.A.; de Carvalho, D.S.; Raboni, S.M.; Shimakura, S.E.; de Mello, A.M.; da Costa-Ribeiro, M.C.V.; Silva, L.; Buffon, M.d.C.M.; Maluf, E.M.C.P.; Graeff, G.; et al. Effectiveness of mass dengue vaccination with CYD-TDV (Dengvaxia®) in the state of Paraná, Brazil: Integrating case-cohort and case-control designs. *Lancet Reg. Health Am.* **2024**, *35*, 100777. [CrossRef]

https://doi.org/10.3390/tropicalmed11010011

8. Ministério da Saúde; Secretaria de Vigilância em Saúde; Departamento de Vigilância Epidemiológica (Eds.) *Sistema de Informação de Agravos de Notificação (Sinan): Normas e Rotinas*, 2nd ed.; Editora do Ministério da Saúde: Brasília, Brasil, 2007; 68p, ISBN 978-85-334-1331-3.
9. Bernal, J.L.; Cummins, S.; Gasparrini, A. Interrupted time series regression for the evaluation of public health interventions: A tutorial. *Int. J. Epidemiol.* **2017**, *46*, 348–355. [CrossRef]
10. Santana, C.P.; Luhm, K.R.; Shimakura, S.E. Impact of Tdap vaccine during pregnancy on the incidence of pertussis in children under one year in Brazil—A time series analysis. *Vaccine* **2021**, *39*, 976–983. [CrossRef]
11. Preto, C.; de Mello, A.M.; Maluf, E.M.C.P.; Krainski, E.T.; Graeff, G.; de Sousa, G.A.; da Silva, L.R.; da Costa-Ribeiro, M.C.V.; Buffon, M.d.C.M.; Shimakura, S.E.; et al. Vaccination coverage and adherence to a dengue vaccination program in the state of Paraná, Brazil. *Vaccine* **2021**, *39*, 711–719. [CrossRef]
12. Dickens, B.L.; Sun, H.; Jit, M.; Cook, A.R.; Carrasco, L.R. Determining environmental and anthropogenic factors which explain the global distribution of *Aedes aegypti* and *Ae. albopictus*. *BMJ Glob. Health* **2018**, *3*, e000801. [CrossRef]
13. Watts, D.M.; Burke, D.S.; Harrison, B.A.; Whitmire, R.E.; Nisalak, A. Effect of temperature on the vector efficiency of *Aedes aegypti* for dengue 2 virus. *Am. J. Trop. Med. Hyg.* **1987**, *36*, 143–152. [CrossRef]
14. Carrington, L.B.; Armijos, M.V.; Lambrechts, L.; Scott, T.W. Fluctuations at a Low Mean Temperature Accelerate Dengue Virus Transmission by *Aedes aegypti*. *PLoS Negl. Trop. Dis.* **2013**, *7*, E2190. [CrossRef]
15. Lambrechts, L.; Paaijmans, K.P.; Fansiri, T.; Carrington, L.B.; Kramer, L.D.; Thomas, M.B.; Scott, T.W. Impact of daily temperature fluctuations on dengue virus transmission by *Aedes aegypti*. *Proc. Natl. Acad. Sci. USA* **2011**, *108*, 7460–7465. [CrossRef] [PubMed]
16. Gomes, A.F.; Nobre, A.A.; Cruz, O.G. Temporal analysis of the relationship between dengue and meteorological variables in the city of Rio de Janeiro, Brazil, 2001–2009. *Cad. Saude Publica* **2012**, *28*, 2189–2197. [CrossRef] [PubMed]
17. Tjaden, N.B.; Thomas, S.M.; Fischer, D.; Beierkuhnlein, C. Extrinsic Incubation Period of Dengue: Knowledge, Backlog, and Applications of Temperature Dependence. *PLoS Negl. Trop. Dis.* **2013**, *7*, e2207. [CrossRef] [PubMed]
18. Lindgren, F.; Rue, H.; Lindström, J. An explicit link between Gaussian fields and Gaussian Markov random fields: The stochastic partial differential equation approach. *J. R. Stat. Soc. Ser. B Stat. Methodol.* **2011**, *7*, 423–498. [CrossRef]
19. Rue, H.; Martino, S.; Chopin, N. Approximate Bayesian inference for latent Gaussian models using integrated nested Laplace approximations (with discussion). *J. R. Stat. Soc.* **2009**, *71*, 19–392. [CrossRef]
20. R Core Team. *R: A Language and Environment for Statistical Computing*; R Foundation for Statistical Computing: Vienna, Austria, 2022.
21. Simpson, D.; Rue, H.; Riebler, A.; Martins, T.G.; Sørbye, S.H. Penalising model component complexity: A principled, practical approach to constructing priors. *Stat. Sci.* **2017**, *32*, 1–28. [CrossRef]
22. Sørbye, S.H.; Rue, H. Penalised Complexity Priors for Stationary Autoregressive Processes. *J. Time Ser. Anal.* **2017**, *38*, 923–935. [CrossRef]
23. Van Niekerk, J.; Rue, H. Correcting the Laplace method with variational Bayes. *arXiv* **2021**, arXiv:2111.12945. [CrossRef]
24. de Souza, S.J.P.; Guaraldo, A.d.C.; Honório, N.A.; Câmara, D.C.P.; Sukow, N.M.; Machado, S.T.; dos Santos, C.N.D.; da Costa-Ribeiro, M.C.V. Spatial and Temporal Distribution of *Aedes aegypti* and *Aedes albopictus* Oviposition on the Coast of Paraná, Brazil, a Recent Area of Dengue Virus Transmission. *Trop. Med. Infect. Dis.* **2022**, *7*, 246. [CrossRef]
25. Halim, N.M.H.N.A.; Dom, N.C.; Dapari, R.; Salim, H.; Precha, N. A systematic review and meta-analysis of the effects of temperature on the development and survival of the *Aedes* mosquito. *Front. Public Health* **2022**, *10*, 1074028. [CrossRef]
26. Leandro, G.C.W.; Cicchelero, L.M.; Procopiuk, M.; Correa, F.d.O.B.; dos Santos, P.C.F.; Lopes, A.R.; Nihei, O.K. Análise temporal e espacial dos casos municipais de dengue no Paraná e indicadores sociais e ambientais, 2012 a 2021: Estudo ecológico. *Rev. Bras. Epidemiol.* **2022**, *25*, e220039. [CrossRef] [PubMed]
27. Drumond, B.P.; Mondini, A.; Schmidt, D.J.; Bosch, I.; Nogueira, M.L. Population dynamics of DENV-1 genotype V in Brazil is characterized by co-circulation and strain/lineage replacement. *Arch. Virol.* **2012**, *157*, 2061–2073. [CrossRef]
28. dos Santos, F.B.; Nogueira, F.B.; Castro, M.G.; Nunes, P.C.; de Filippis, A.M.B.; Faria, N.R.; Simões, J.B.; A Sampaio, S.; Santos, C.R.; Nogueira, R.M.R. First report of multiple lineages of dengue viruses type 1 in Rio de Janeiro, Brazil. *Virol. J.* **2011**, *8*, 387. [CrossRef] [PubMed]
29. Bezerra, J.M.T.; de Sousa, S.C.; Tauil, P.L.; Carneiro, M.; Barbosa, D.S. Entry of dengue virus serotypes and their geographic distribution in Brazilian federative units: A systematic review. *Rev. Bras. Epidemiol.* **2021**, *24*, e210020. [CrossRef] [PubMed]
30. Rodriguez-Barraquer, I.; Cordeiro, M.T.; Braga, C.; de Souza, W.V.; Marques, E.T.; Cummings, D.A.T. From re-emergence to hyperendemicity: The natural history of the dengue epidemic in Brazil. *PLoS Negl. Trop. Dis.* **2011**, *5*, e935. [CrossRef]
31. Nunes, P.C.G.; Daumas, R.P.; Sánchez-Arcila, J.C.; Nogueira, R.M.R.; Horta, M.A.P.; dos Santos, F.B. 30 years of fatal dengue cases in Brazil: A review. *BMC Public Health* **2019**, *19*, 329. [CrossRef]
32. de Castro, D.B.; Sampaio, V.S.; de Albuquerque, B.C.; Pinto, R.C.; Sadahiro, M.; dos Passos, R.A.; da Costa, C.F.; Braga, J.U. Dengue epidemic typology and risk factors for extensive epidemic in Amazonas state, Brazil, 2010–2011. *BMC Public Health* **2018**, *18*, 356. [CrossRef]

 https://doi.org/10.3390/tropicalmed11010011

33. Yang, X.; Quam, M.B.M.; Zhang, T.; Sang, S. Global burden for dengue and the evolving pattern in the past 30 years. *J. Travel Med.* **2021**, *28*, taab146. [CrossRef]
34. Guy, B.; Briand, O.; Lang, J.; Saville, M.; Jackson, N. Development of the Sanofi Pasteur tetravalent dengue vaccine: One more step forward. *Vaccine* **2015**, *33*, 7100–7111. [CrossRef]
35. Luhm, K.R.; Shimakura, S.E.; Raboni, S.M.; da Costa-Ribeiro, M.C.V.; Diaz-Quijano, F.A.; de Mello, A.M.; Silva, L.; Buffon, M.d.C.M.; Maluf, E.M.C.P.; Graeff, G.; et al. Dengue Vaccine Effectiveness: Results from a 6-Year Population-Based Cohort Study in Southern Brazil. *Am. J. Trop. Med. Hyg.* 2025; ahead of print. [CrossRef]

https://doi.org/10.3390/tropicalmed11010011

Tropical Medicine and Infectious Disease

MDPI

Article

Limited Spectroscopy Data and Machine Learning for Detection of Zika Virus Infection in *Aedes aegypti* Mosquitoes

Leonardo Reigoto [1], Rafael Maciel-de-Freitas [2,3,*], Maggy T. Sikulu-Lord [4,5], Gabriela A. Garcia [2], Gabriel Araujo [6] and Amaro Lima [7]

1 Universidade Federal Fluminense, Niteroi 24220-900, RJ, Brazil; lreigoto@id.uff.br
2 Laboratório de Mosquitos Transmissores de Hematozoários, Instituto Oswaldo Cruz, Rio de Janeiro 21040-360, RJ, Brazil; gabiazambuja@hotmail.com
3 Department of Entomology and Arbovirology, Bernhard Nocht Institute for Tropical Medicine, 20359 Hamburg, Germany
4 School of the Environment, Faculty of Science, The University of Queensland, Brisbane, QLD 4072, Australia; maggy.lord@uq.edu.au
5 NIRSID Consortium, Brisbane, QLD 4072, Australia
6 Program of Electrical Engineering, Federal Centre of Technological Education of Rio de Janeiro (CEFET/RJ), Campus Maracanã, Rio de Janeiro 20911-020, RJ, Brazil; gabriel.araujo@cefet-rj.br
7 Program of Instrumentation and Applied Optics, Federal Centre of Technological Education of Rio de Janeiro (CEFET/RJ), Campus Maracanã, Rio de Janeiro 20911-020, RJ, Brazil; amaro.lima@cefet-rj.br
* Correspondence: freitas@ioc.fiocruz.br or macieldefreitas@bnitm.de; Tel.: +55-21-99927-0481

Abstract

This study presents a technique for categorizing *Aedes aegypti* mosquitoes infected with the Zika virus under laboratory conditions. Our approach involves the utilization of the near-infrared spectroscopy technique and machine learning algorithms. The model developed utilizes the absorption of light from 350 to 1000 nm. It integrates Linear Discriminant Analysis (LDA) of the signal's windowed version to exploit non-linearities, along with Support Vector Machine (SVM) for classification purposes. Our proposed methodology can identify the presence of the Zika virus in intact mosquitoes with a balanced accuracy of 96% (row C2HT, average of columns TPR (%) and SPC (%)) when heads/thoraces of mosquitoes are scanned at 4, 7, and 10 days post virus infection. The model was 97.1% (10 DPI, row C2AB, column ACC (%)) accurate for mosquitoes that were used to test it, i.e., mosquitoes scanned 10-days post-infection and mosquitoes whose abdomens were scanned. Notable benefits include its cost-effectiveness and the capability for real-time predictions. This work also demonstrates the role played by different spectral wavelengths in predicting an infection in mosquitoes.

Keywords: Zika virus; machine learning; detection; arboviruses; classification; Support Vector Machine

1. Introduction

Among the diverse group of arboviruses, certain pathogens such as dengue virus (DENV), Zika virus (ZIKV), and chikungunya virus (CHIKV) have emerged as significant global public health concerns due to their pathogenic potential and capacity to trigger explosive outbreaks in densely populated urban environments [1–3]. The primary vector responsible for the transmission of these arboviruses is *Aedes aegypti*, a mosquito species highly adapted to urban ecosystems. *Aedes aegypti* exhibits a strong anthropophilic behavior, preferentially feeding on human blood, and commonly oviposits in artificial water-holding containers located in or near human dwellings. Its limited dispersal range is typically restricted to a few hundred meters which further reinforces its close association with domestic and peridomestic habitats [4–9].

Given the rapid and unpredictable nature of arbovirus transmission, the effectiveness of vector control strategies hinges on the implementation of robust and timely entomological surveillance systems [10,11]. Surveillance programs based on the systematic sampling of immature and adult mosquito populations provide critical insights into vector abundance and spatial distribution, serving as the foundation for evidence-based public health decision-making [12–16]. However, conventional surveillance methods often suffer from limitations in spatial resolution and operational efficiency, necessitating refinement to meet contemporary demands [14,17,18].

To enhance vector control outcomes, mosquito surveillance data should be integrated into spatial and temporal analytical frameworks capable of generating dynamic risk maps [10,19–21]. These models can identify intra-urban transmission hotspots, enabling geographically targeted interventions that maximize resource allocation and operational impact. In this context, integrated vector management (IVM) strategies that align entomological surveillance with tailored control measures represent a promising paradigm for sustainable arbovirus control [22,23]. Ultimately, refined surveillance systems not only support epidemic preparedness and response but also facilitate continuous monitoring of disease trends, evaluation of intervention efficacy, and adaptive management of vector control programs. Such approaches empower local public health authorities to optimize control efforts and mitigate arboviral disease burden more effectively [24].

Recent advances in mathematical modeling and computational methods have significantly contributed to understanding and predicting mosquito-borne diseases such as dengue and Zika. Jose et al. (2024) conducted a comprehensive study on dengue incidence in Thailand, applying statistical and machine learning approaches—including exponential smoothing, polynomial fitting, and Random Forest models—to forecast outbreak dynamics and enhance public health preparedness [25]. In a complementary framework, Jose et al. (2023) developed a deterministic model describing the co-infection dynamics of Zika virus and dengue fever, highlighting through bifurcation and stability analyses the intricate interactions between human hosts and mosquito vectors [26]. From a biological control perspective, Joseph et al. (2023) proposed a fractional-order, density-dependent model to evaluate the dissemination of different Wolbachia strains in *Aedes aegypti* populations, identifying the wAlbB strain as the most effective in suppressing viral transmission [27]. Together, these studies demonstrate the potential of quantitative and data-driven approaches for understanding arboviral transmission and guiding vector control strategies. Building upon this foundation, the present study explores the integration of spectroscopy data and machine learning techniques as an innovative diagnostic approach for detecting Zika virus infection in *Aedes aegypti* mosquitoes, particularly under conditions of limited or sparse spectral information.

Zika virus (ZIKV), a member of the *Flaviviridae* family, was historically considered a geographically constrained and poorly characterized pathogen, primarily circulating in specific regions of Africa. However, in the early 2010s, ZIKV expanded its geographical range, culminating in a major outbreak in South America. In 2015, its association with severe neurological outcomes—such as congenital microcephaly in neonates and Guillain–Barré syndrome in adults—led the World Health Organization to designate it a Public Health Emergency of International Concern [28–31]. Although ZIKV transmission has declined globally following this epidemic, it remains an important model for studying the epidemiology and control of emerging and re-emerging mosquito-borne diseases. Effective surveillance of ZIKV, as with other arboviruses, requires surveillance tools that are not only sensitive and specific but also scalable, cost-effective, and operationally feasible for large-scale field deployment. Molecular diagnostic tools such as polymerase chain reaction (PCR) and quantitative PCR (qPCR) have long been the gold standard for detecting arboviral RNA in mosquito vectors [32]. Nevertheless, the logistical demands of these techniques—particularly their reliance on expensive reagents, skilled personnel, and time-consuming protocols—pose substantial barriers to widespread implementation in routine entomological surveillance. In response to these challenges, near-infrared spectroscopy (NIRS) has emerged as a promising alternative diagnostic modality. NIRS operates within a wavelength range of approximately 750–2500 nm and quantifies the absorption of light by specific chemical bonds (e.g., C–H, O–H, S–H, and N–H) within a biological sample [33,34]. The resulting spectral signatures reflect the molecular composition of the sample and can be analyzed to infer key biological parameters. This technique offers several operational advantages: it is non-destructive (preserving the sample for future analyses), reagent-free (minimizing costs), rapid (yielding results in seconds), and environmentally sustainable (generating no chemical waste) [35].

Researchers have previously utilized NIRS within the wavelength range of 700 to 2500 nm to identify the presence of the Zika virus in mosquitoes [36]. The obtained spectra were mean-centered and then subjected to classification through the Partial Least Squares (PLS) regression technique in GRAMS Plus/IQ software from Thermo Galactic. The outcomes of this method are presented in Table 1.

Table 1. NIRS method [36], where C1TR stands for Cohort 1 train, C1VS for Cohort 1 validation (sorted), C2HT for Cohort 2 head/thorax, C2AB for Cohort 2 abdomen, TPR for True Positive Rate, SPC for specificity, and DPI for days post infection.

Dataset	4 DPI		7 DPI		10 DPI	
	TPR (%)	SPC (%)	TPR (%)	SPC (%)	TPR (%)	SPC (%)
C1TR	83.3	96.8	93.5	96.4	-	-
C1VS	100.0	94.1	100.0	100.0	-	-
C2HT	98.7	98.3	100.0	98.3	100.0	86.7
C2AB	98.7	85.0	96.2	80.0	97.4	68.3

The primary issue with the approach outlined in [36] lies in its cost. Acquiring a near-infrared spectrograph can entail expenses running into the thousands of dollars. This study seeks to explore the feasibility of detecting the Zika virus in mosquitoes using a narrower band of wavelengths while leveraging advanced machine learning algorithms. Specifically, we apply Linear Discriminant Analysis (LDA) and Support Vector Machine (SVM) to the dataset from [36], focusing solely on wavelengths between 350 and 1000 nm. It is worth mentioning that other techniques, such as Principal Component Analysis (PCA) and Random Forest (RF), were also evaluated, but the most effective combination was the use of LDA and SVM. From a financial standpoint, a comprehensive near-infrared spectrometer (covering 350 to 2500 nm, which corresponds to the last part of ultraviolet, UV, the whole visible, VIS, and the whole near-infrared, NIR, spectra) typically carries a price tag around US $60,000 (LabSpec 4i NIR spectrometer acquired and used in this work). In contrast, certain spectrometers capable of detecting light within the 350 to 1000 nm range can be found for around US $1500 (the model investigated was ATP1000−UV-VIS-NIR-5 from optosky.com). Electrochemical technology [37], with an estimated cost of tens of dollars, which identifies dengue and Zika viruses in solutions, cannot replace the spectrometer approach for this work, due to the fact that the conditions of applicability of the two technologies are quite different. For example, one requires a solution of the virus and the other requires the intact body of the mosquito. The main achievement of this work is to show that applying discriminative and classification techniques in a narrower spectral bandwidth could provide equivalent performance to the whole spectral bandwidth available in this work for identifying the Zika virus in intact mosquitoes, possibly reducing the implementation cost. The structure of this paper is as follows: Section 2 provides an overview of the dataset initially introduced in [36] and utilized in this study. Section 3 delves into the proposed methodology. Section 4 presents the obtained results and a subsequent discussion. Concluding remarks can be found in Section 5.

2. Dataset

The dataset utilized in this research was built and obtained from [36]. This dataset encompasses three key variables:

- The absorbance measurements at various wavelengths, ranging from 350 to 2500 nm;
- The infection status of the mosquito (infected or uninfected);
- The duration measured in days post infection (DPI).

In Figure 1, a comparison of absorbance versus wavelength is presented for two distinct samples. The blue line represents an uninfected mosquito, whereas the orange line denotes an infected mosquito (7 DPI). It also presents three sensor ranges used in the spectrometer, silicon (350 to 1000 nm) and InGaAs sensors (sensor 1: 1000 to 1800 nm, and sensor 2: 1800 to 2500 nm), along with the UV, VIS, and NIR limits.

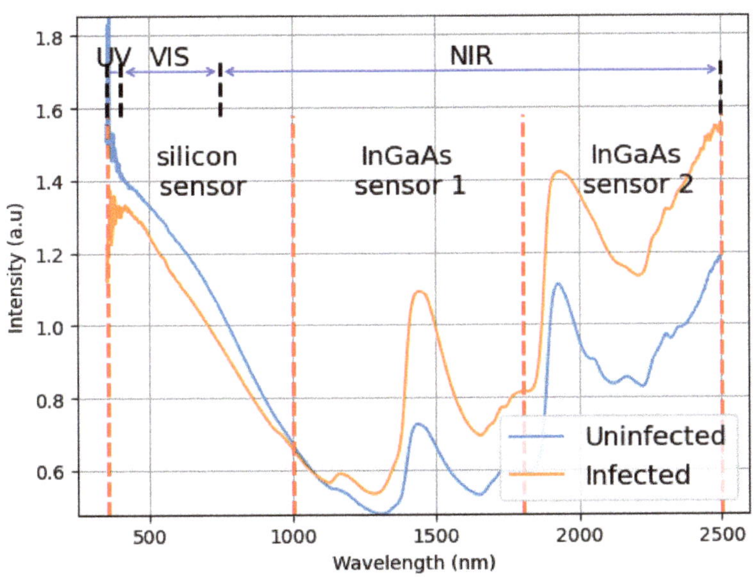

Figure 1. Example of the difference between the average spectrum of the mosquitoes infected and non-infected. This graph plots the result of the spectroscopy (intensity of light) versus the measured wavelengths (350 to 2500 nm). It also shows the ranges of the three sensors used in the equipment, silicon (350 to 1000 nm), and InGaAs (sensor 1: 1000 to 1800 nm, and sensor 2: 1800 to 2500 nm) sensors and how they are related to UV (350 to 400 nm), VIS (400 to 750 nm) and NIR (750 to 2500 nm).

In this experiment, we utilized female *Ae. aegypti* mosquitoes that were either 5 or 6 days old when they received their first blood meal. Briefly, an infective blood meal containing human blood from an anonymous donor and Zika virus was offered to half of the mosquitoes reared under standard conditions (27 ± 2 °C, 70 ± 5 relative humidity). The other half received ZIKV-uninfected blood from the same donor, plus C6/36 cell culture instead of virus. We established two distinct cohorts of mosquitoes, each collected and measured independently, with scans collected at 4, 7, and 10 days post infection (DPI). Prior to taking measurements, the mosquitoes were immobilised by placing them in a sealed jar with a cotton ball soaked in ethyl acetate for 1 min. Subsequently, a NIRS spectrometer was employed to analyze the absorbance across a range of wavelengths from 350 to 2500 nm, utilizing the LabSpec 4i NIR spectrometer from Malvern Panalytical, which features an internal 18.6 W light source.

For Cohort 1, spectra were collected from the head/thorax of the mosquitoes. For Cohort 2 two separate spectra were collected as follows: spectra of the combined head/thorax and spectra of the abdomen. Following these measurements, RT-qPCR tests were conducted on infected mosquitoes to confirm infection.

Samples from each cohort were classified according to DPI (4, 7, and 10) and infection status (infected and not infected), resulting in up to six groups for each cohort, as illustrated in Figures 2 and 3.

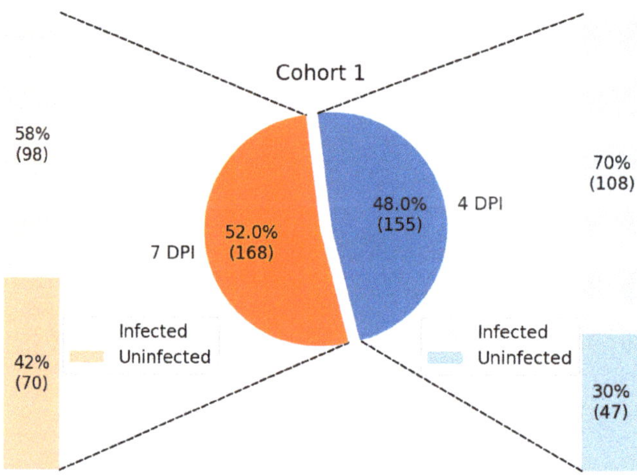

Figure 2. Distribution of samples from Cohort 1, training dataset, shown in percentage and with its respective number of samples enclosed in parenthesis.

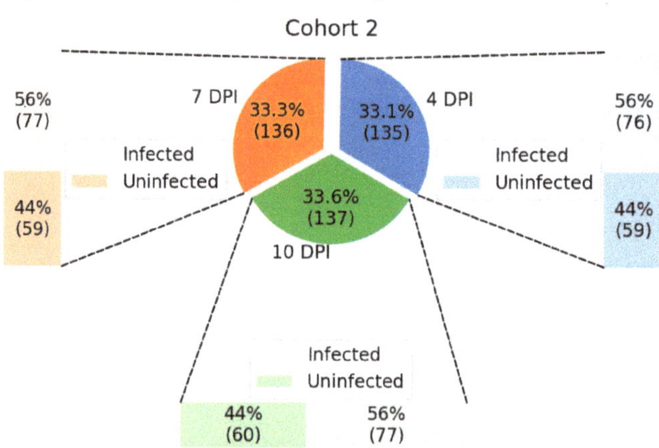

Figure 3. Distribution of samples from Cohort 2, test dataset, shown in percentage and with its respective number of samples enclosed in parenthesis.

The data from Cohort 1 contains (a) 108 infected samples and 47 uninfected samples at 4 DPI; and (b) 98 infected samples and 70 uninfected samples at 7 DPI, making a total of 323 samples.

The data from Cohort 2 contains: (a) 76 infected samples and 59 uninfected samples at 4 DPI; (b) 77 infected samples and 59 uninfected samples at 7 DPI; and (c) 77 infected samples and 60 uninfected samples at 10 DPI, having 408 samples in total.

The spectrometer used combines three devices: (1) a silicon sensor that operates between 350 and 1000 nm; (2) an InGaAs sensor that operates between 1001 and 1800 nm; and (3) an InGaAs sensor that operates between 1801 and 2500 nm. Our model was designed using only the readings from the first device (the silicon sensor), as this wavelenght is most commonly found in low-cost equipment. However, a comprehensive comparison of efficiency among the other sensors data was also carried out.

3. Methodology

In this paper, we utilized samples from Cohort 1 to train our model and subsequently tested the model with data from Cohort 2, which can be considered unseen in the sense that it was not used in the training. This approach provides the benefit of having training and testing data that were collected and measured independently. Given that the preparation of mosquitoes and the associated measurements can be quite intricate, this separation of data aids in ensuring that our model can generalize effectively and predict the status of new samples rather than merely fitting to noise present in the data.

There are two issues concerning the remaining data: its limited number of samples and its high dimensionality. While excluding samples from Cohort 2 from our training data exacerbates the challenges posed by the scarcity of data, the benefits of this approach outweigh the drawbacks. It is essential to demonstrate that our model can generalize effectively. We employed the k-fold method ($k = 10$) to validate our model using samples from Cohort 1 without the necessity of removing them from our training dataset. Note that the validation data is part of the whole training data, Cohort 1. It is related to k-fold and used to find the hyperparameters associated to the most efficient k-fold model, which are used in the learning process of the whole training data generating a single model. The test data, Cohort 2, is related to the model evaluation.

The k-fold method involves partitioning the data into k distinct folds. We then trained our model k times, each time excluding one fold from the training data and utilizing it for model evaluation. The final evaluation metrics are derived from the average of all k models and the final model is a synthesis of all individual models. In classification tasks, the predicted class can be determined by the majority vote among all models. It is a common practice to assess a model using k-fold validation to find out the best hyperparameters associated the highest accurate k-fold model, which are subsequently used to create a new single model by training on all folds, i.e., on the whole training data, Cohort 2. If we obtain a sufficient quantity of data and folds to minimize noise from specific samples, it is anticipated, according to the theory of generalization [38] that our final model will closely resemble the amalgamation of the original k models.

3.1. Applying LDA

To address the dimensionality issue, we eliminated data that contributes minimal information. Our dataset, which consists of absorbance measurements against wavelength, was expected to reveal some level of linearity since the data is being classified over a continuous range. This property allowed us to utilize Linear Discriminant Analysis (LDA) [39,40] as a feature extractor, effectively handling dimensionality challenges. LDA works by transforming the axes of our parameters into new dimensions that enhance class discrimination.

Its primary objective is to identify a projection axis that maximizes the variance between classes while minimizing the variance within each class. By transforming the data in this way, it became possible to distinguish between classes using fewer parameters, which means we could confidently discard some of the original data elements. For a visual comparison, see Figure 4, which illustrates the spectral band from 350 to 1000 nm for both infected and non-infected mosquitoes.

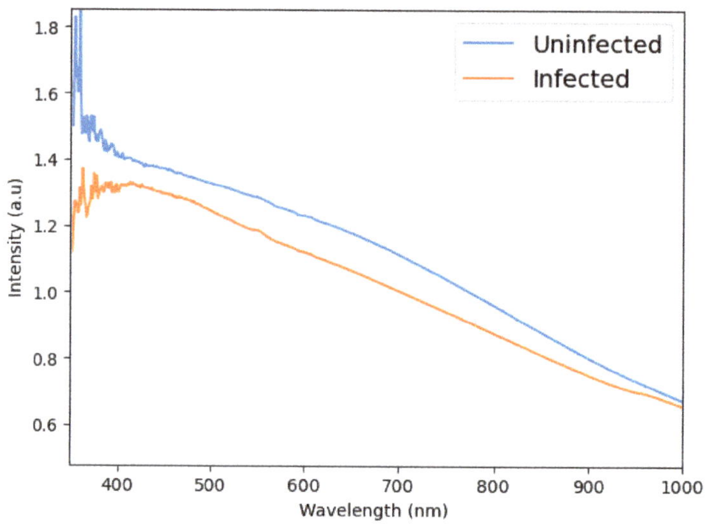

Figure 4. Example of the difference between the average spectrum of the mosquitoes infected and not-infected with ZIKV. This graph plots the result of the spectroscopy (intensity of light) versus the measured wavelengths (350 to 1000 nm).

The idea behind LDA is to transform our parameter axes in new ones that best discriminate our classes. The main focus of the LDA is to separate the classes by jointly maximizing the distance between their centers and minimizing the variance of each individually. This concept can be seen in Figure 5, where a new axis that indicates an optimization towards the discrimination between the classes is generated.

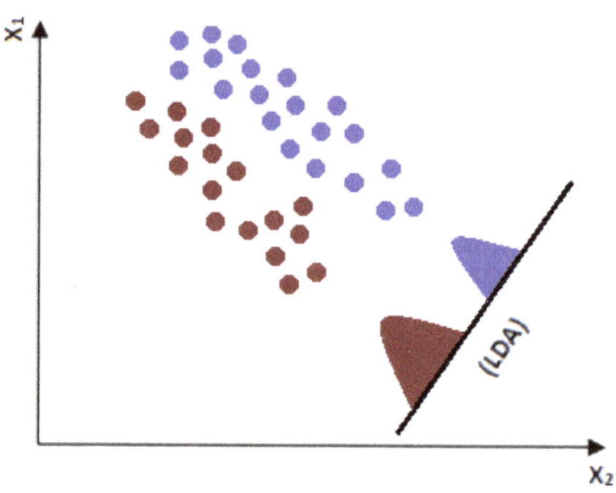

Figure 5. Illustrative example of a new axis generated by LDA.

We employed the LDA algorithm to derive new features from our dataset. In classification scenarios involving C classes, the LDA algorithm yields $C-1$ axes that most effectively differentiate the classes. Given that the current problem only encompasses 2 classes (infected or not), the LDA algorithm produced merely 1 axis. Consequently, our model could only identify a threshold line along this axis and classify based on that threshold. A limitation of this method is its inability to address non-linearity, which could enhance the algorithm's effectiveness. To overcome this limitation, we selected a reduced wavelength range of $(350, 1000]$ nm, corresponding to the ith intensity vector $\mathbf{x}_i = [x(1), \ldots, x(650)]$, and partitioned it into twenty-six non-overlapping windows, each with intervals of 25 wavelengths, resulting in ranges of $(350, 375]$, ..., $(975, 1000]$ nm. We generated LDA models for each window's associated data, denoted as $\text{LDA}_1, \ldots, \text{LDA}_{26}$, plus one more LDA model obtained from the entire interval, denoted as LDA_{all}, and applied the vector window to its corresponding LDA coordinates, thereby producing the projection of the vector window in LDA space. The twenty-seven projections were concatenated to form the feature vector, $[x'_1, \ldots, x'_{26}, x'_{\text{all}}]$. This vector consists of an axis that optimally discriminates each vector window plus the entire interval. Each axis can still be utilized to classify each window plus the whole interval based on a threshold, but they can also indicate the reliability of these classifications through the distance from the threshold.

After obtaining the feature vector by concatenating the projections from LDA, we utilized a Support Vector Machine (SVM) for data classification, which yields the output y_i corresponding to $\mathbf{x}_i$. The entire system, named as LDA + SVM, can be seen in Figure 6, showing the training and test sets are performed using Cohort 1 and Cohort 2 datasets, respectively. The LDA models for feature extraction used in test phase are the same generated during the training.

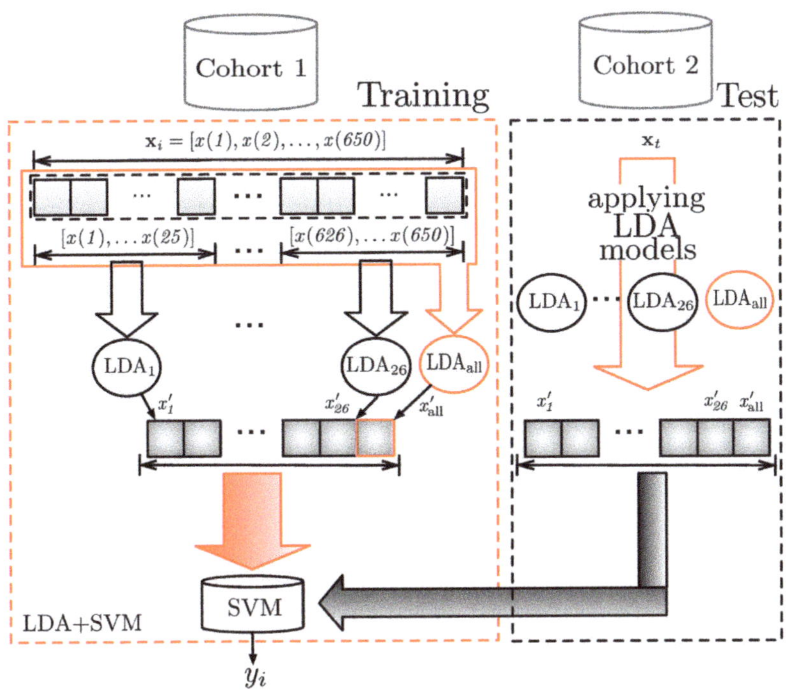

Figure 6. Block diagram of LDA + SVM approach and training and test setups.

3.2. *SVM for Classification*

The Support Vector Machine (SVM) [41–44] is an exceptionally powerful and widely utilized algorithm. It has the capability to replicate the outcomes of more complex models while utilizing simpler ones. This characteristic enables the algorithm to manage a greater number of parameters with a reduced amount of data, demonstrating increased resilience against the *curse of dimensionality* [42] and *overfitting*.

The fundamental concept of SVM involves utilizing the hyperspace of input parameters to identify the optimal hyperplane that separates two classes. This hyperplane is designed to maximize the margin between the classes, which is determined by the support vectors. Support vectors are the data points that lie on the margin of the hyperplane. Furthermore, this margin classifier is capable of addressing non-linearly separable classes by transforming the data into a higher-dimensional space ϕ, which is practically executed through kernel functions, with the most prevalent being polynomial and radial basis kernels. We utilized the new vector generated from the LDA algorithms as input for a Support Vector Machine (SVM) with a polynomial kernel. By employing a non-linear kernel, our model gains additional complexity. The SVM aims to identify the hyperplane that best separates the data. As previously mentioned, our new vector represents the projection of each window along the axis that distinguishes it most effectively while also conveying the reliability of each discriminant. Essentially, the SVM aligns with the geometric structure of our data.

4. Results

The experimental results were generated by applying the proposed LDA + SVM system in the restricted wavelength range of 350 to 1000 nm for all subsets of the whole dataset (training and test), considering all different DPIs, and the composite performance using five evaluation metrics commonly applied to classification problems. A performance comparison between the three sensor ranges represented in the dataset plus the VIS spectrum was also evaluated. This second part of the results considered only the test set. The findings from the LDA + SVM approach considering the wavelength range from 350 to 1000 nm can be found in Tables 2 and 3.

Table 2. LDA + SVM (350 to 1000 nm) stratified in 4, 7, and 10 DPI, where C1TR stands for Cohort 1 train, C1VS for Cohort 1 *k*-fold validation, C2HT for Cohort 2 head/thorax, and C2AB for Cohort 2 abdomen, where TPR, SPC, PRC, ACC, F1S, are True Positive Rate, Specificity, Precision, Accuracy, F1-Score, respectively.

Dataset	TPR (%)	SPC (%)	PRC (%)	ACC (%)	F1S (%)
			4 DPI		
C1TR	100.0	100.0	100.0	100.0	100.0
C1VS	100.0 ± 0.0	93.5 ± 10.3	96.5 ± 6.3	97.6 ± 4.2	98.1 ± 3.5
C2HT	100.0	86.4	90.5	94.1	95.0
C2AB	100.0	95.0	96.2	97.8	98.1
			7 DPI		
C1TR	100.0	100.0	100.0	100.0	100.0
C1VS	100.0 ± 0.0	93.7 ± 9.6	94.8 ± 7.9	96.9 ± 4.8	97.2 ± 4.3
C2HT	100	93.2	95.1	97.1	97.5
C2AB	94.8	100	100	97.1	97.3

Table 2. *Cont.*

Dataset	TPR (%)	SPC (%)	PRC (%)	ACC (%)	F1S (%)
			10 DPI		
C1TR	-	-	-	-	-
C1VS	-	-	-	-	-
C2HT	98.7	98.3	98.7	98.5	98.7
C2AB	94.8	100	100	97.1	97.3

Table 3. LDA + SVM (350 to 1000 nm) with no DPI stratification, where C1TR stands for Cohort 1 train, C1VS for Cohort 1 *k*-fold validation, C2HT for Cohort 2 head/thorax, and C2AB for Cohort 2 abdomen, where TPR, SPC, PRC, ACC, F1S, are True Positive Rate, Specificity, Precision, Accuracy, F1-Score, respectively.

			No DPI Stratification (%)		
Dataset	**TPR (%)**	**SPC (%)**	**PRC (%)**	**ACC (%)**	**F1S (%)**
C1TR	100.0	100.0	100.0	100.0	100.0
C1VS	100.0 ± 0.0	91.8 ± 7.2	95.3 ± 4.3	96.9 ± 2.8	97.5 ± 2.2
C2HT	99.6	92.7	94.6	96.6	97.0
C2AB	98.3	96.7	97.4	97.6	97.8

Table 2 presents the stratified results from the metrics True Positive Rate (TPR), also known as Recall and Sensitivity, Specificity (SPC), Precision (PRC), Accuracy (ACC), and F1-Score (F1S). Comparing the results displayed in Tables 1 and 2, i.e., comparing two different models, it is observed that the proposed method attained a better TPR, which means a lower number of false negatives (FN) in almost all cases, except for C2HT at 10 DPI and C2AB at 7 and 10 DPI. However, considering the balanced accuracy $\left(\frac{\text{TPR}+\text{SPC}}{2}\right)$ in these three exceptions, the proposed method performed better, representing a certain balance between the percentages of true positives (TP) and true negatives (TN) within the actual classes. It is worth noting that a lower FN means the error of predicting infected mosquito as uninfected is reduced. Applying the same rationale, the SPC in the three exceptional cases is higher in the proposed method, meaning that the number of false positives (FPs) is lower, which represents a higher percentage of truly infected among all infected predictions. One important remark is that the model was trained without mosquitoes at 10 DPI, so this group of mosquitoes with higher balanced accuracy indicates a good generalized model, which can also be confirmed by observing the ACC metric for the C2HT dataset at 4 and 7 DPI, reaching 94.1% and 97.1%, respectively, and for the C2AB dataset at 4, 7, and 10 DPI, reaching 97.8%, 97.1%, and 97.1%, respectively. These results indicate generalization not only in unseen data but also in data without representation in training.

Table 2, row C2HT, column ACC (%) achieves 94.1% and 97.1% for 4 and 7 DPI, respectively. Also observing the same Table 2, row C2AB, column ACC (%) achieve 97.8% and 97.1% for 4 and 7 DPI, respectively. Furthermore, the same row and column for 10 DPI achieves 97.1%.

Table 3 presents the same results of Table 1 without DPI stratification, which is the statistics to be considered whenever this approach is applied in a field situation. For datasets C2HT and C2AB, no metric was lower than 92%, while the metrics TPR and F1S reached over 97%. Comparing the metrics in the same model, TPR values were higher than PRC with over 94%, indicating that the number of FP is higher than FN, and that the proposed model is more likely to find an infected mosquito than to miss it.

In order to analyze the proposed approach in different wavelength ranges, an experiment was devised applying the LDA + SVM method to the spectrum range concerning the original spectrometer silicon sensor from 350 to 1000 nm, InGaAs sensor 1 from 1000 to 1800 nm, and sensor 2 from 1800 to 2500 nm. In addition to that, the visible spectrum range, from 400 to 750 nm, was also added to the experiment. The results are presented in Table 4 for the test datasets C2HT and C2AB encompassing all the metrics (TPR, SPC, PRC, ACC, and F1S) with no DPI stratification. It can be noticed that the range originally chosen to develop the proposed model hit the higher performance in all metrics, probably because this spectrum range carries the most discriminative information to fulfill the task.

Table 4. Comparing different wavelength ranges associated to the original spectrometer sensors (350–1000 nm, 1001–1800 nm, and 1801–2500 nm) and visible light (400–750 nm) without classifying mosquitoes into DPI for test datasets within Cohort 2 for head/thorax scans and within Cohort 2 for abdomen using TPR, SPC, PRC, ACC, and F1S metrics.

Range (nm)	TPR (%)	SPC (%)	PRC (%)	ACC (%)	F1S (%)
		Cohort 2 Head/Thorax			
350–1000	99.6	92.7	94.6	96.6	97.0
1001–1800	90.4	41.6	66.7	69.1	76.8
1801–2500	98.3	36.0	66.5	71.1	79.3
400–750 (VIS)	93.5	88.2	91.1	91.2	92.3
		Cohort 2 Abdomen			
350–1000	98.3	96.7	97.4	97.6	97.8
1001–1800	84.3	37.8	63.4	63.9	72.4
1801–2500	97.4	52.2	72.3	77.6	83.0
400–750 (VIS)	97.4	75.6	83.6	87.8	90.0

The second best range in terms of performance was the visible light, which showed higher predictive accuracy compared to InGaAs sensors 1 and 2 ranges, except for TPR in the range from 1800 to 2500 nm for both datasets. However, it was better than the InGaAs sensor 2 in both exceptions considering the balanced accuracy. Commercial instruments comprising the range of the silicon sensor and VIS are the cheapest available options with an average price of US $1500, while the InGaAs sensors 1 and 2 can cost up to US $32,000 (the models investigated were L/300-1100, L/400-740, N/900-1700, and N/900-2500 on simtrum.com). It is worth remembering that the proposed model, LDA + SVM model, was not trained with 10 DPI data nor abdomen measurements, i.e., the model was built without knowing any 10 DPI and abdomen data samples; however, it achieved performance above approximately 95% in these data strata.

5. Conclusions

The findings from this research indicate that it is feasible to detect Zika virus-infected mosquitoes using limited spectral data. This approach could potentially be executed with a more affordable device compared to the traditional Labspec spectrometer. As a result, it opens the door for the development of a budget-friendly IoT solution that can be utilized effectively in the field and improve surveillance of vector-borne diseases.

Reverse Transcription quantitative polymerase chain reaction (RT-qPCR) and standard PCR are the traditional technique for virus detection in mosquitoes [24,32,35]. However, it comes with several drawbacks: it is quite expensive, particularly for large-scale programs that require the analysis of thousands of samples, and it is time consuming and requires skilled personnel to operate. On the other hand, although it can be automated to provide results in real-time, the traditional NIR spectrometer currently in use for mosquito characterization (Labspec 4i) measures wavelengths from 350 to 2500 nm and requires more than US $60,000 as an overlay cost for a spectrometer. These drawbacks limit its applicability in many field settings. Our findings indicate smaller instruments with a smaller band width provide similar results as the traditional benchtop instruments. This is consistent with Takahashi and colleagues' recent findings that demonstrated that a miniaturized spectrometer (NIRvascan) with wavelengths from 900–1700 nm is comparable to the LabSpec instrument for age grading and predicting mosquito blood feeding history [45]. Our findings suggest that a spectrometer with wavelengths from 350 to 1000 nm will provide similar results for detecting viruses in mosquitoes. Although cheaper spectrometers may have lower SNR, raising doubts about the noise robustness of the proposed system, the conclusion of [45] indicates equivalent discriminatory capacity of real data using cheaper equipment compared to more expensive ones.

The proposed LDA + SVM method demonstrated superior generalization in the classification of mosquitoes at 10 DPI when compared to the original approach examined in this study. The data for mosquitoes at 10 DPI and abdomen measurements are considered unseen, as they were not used during the training phase. The addition analysis of different ranges concluded that the VIS region on its own achieved slightly lower predictive accuracy than the range from 350 to 1000 nm, although the commercial equipment have similar costs. The key takeaway is that the proposed method achieves performance levels comparable to those reported in [36], while utilizing significantly less wavelength information.

Given the challenges associated with capturing and infecting mosquitoes, our training dataset is limited in sample size. To enhance the reliability of the statistical information, it is advisable to expand the dataset, preferably incorporating sampling infected and uninfected mosquitoes at different time points post-infection. This approach is expected to yield a more effective training model and potentially improve the accuracy of the system.

Further investigation into hyperparameter optimization and the removal of outliers is a logical next step, as the data has not been thoroughly explored. Future endeavors will also involve the development of a cost-effective IoT device to facilitate these readings and to implement our model in the field.

Author Contributions: Conceptualization, R.M.-d.-F., M.T.S.-L. and G.A.G.; methodology and investigation, A.L. and G.A.; software and investigation, L.R. All authors have read and agreed to the published version of the manuscript.

Funding: We would like to thank Fundação Carlos Chagas Filho de Amparo a Pesquisa no Estado do Rio de Janeiro (E-26/201.075/2002), and Conselho Nacional de Desenvolvimento Científico e Tecnológico (306111/2024-1).

Institutional Review Board Statement: We declare there is no need at all to submit this manuscript to an Institutional Ethical Board. Since we did not handle animal samples. We only used the raw infrared spectral data produced by Fernandes et al. 2018 (available at DOI: 10.1126/sciadv.aat0496) and listed as Reference [36].

Informed Consent Statement: Not applicable.

Data Availability Statement: The data set generated in this paper is available from the corresponding author on reasonable request.

Acknowledgments: The authors would like to thank the following Brazilian Agencies CAPES, CNPq, and FAPERJ.

Conflicts of Interest: The authors declare no conflicts of interest.

References

1. Huang, Y.J.S.; Higgs, S.; Vanlandingham, D.L. Emergence and re-emergence of mosquito-borne arboviruses. *Curr. Opin. Virol.* **2019**, *34*, 104–109. [CrossRef]
2. Weaver, S.C.; Reisen, W.K. Present and future arboviral threats. *Antivir. Res.* **2010**, *85*, 328–345. [CrossRef]
3. Weaver, S.C.; Charlier, C.; Vasilakis, N.; Lecuit, M. Zika, Chikungunya, and Other Emerging Vector-Borne Viral Diseases. *Annu. Rev. Med.* **2018**, *69*, 395–408. [CrossRef] [PubMed]
4. Harrington, L.C.; Scott, T.W.; Lerdthusnee, K.; Coleman, R.C.; Costero, A.; Clark, G.G.; Jones, J.J.; Kitthawee, S.; Kittayapong, P.; Sithiprasasna, R.; et al. Dispersal of the dengue vector Aedes aegypti within and between rural communities. *Am. J. Trop. Med. Hyg.* **2005**, *72*, 209–220. [CrossRef] [PubMed]
5. Maciel-de Freitas, R.; Lourenço-de Oliveira, R. Presumed unconstrained dispersal of Aedes aegypti in the city of Rio de Janeiro. *Rev. Saúde Pública* **2009**, *43*, 8–12. [CrossRef] [PubMed]
6. Maciel-de-Freitas, R.; Codeço, C.T.; de Oliveira, R.L. Daily survival rates and dispersal of Aedes aegypti females in Rio de Janeiro, Brazil. *Am. J. Trop. Med. Hyg.* **2007**, *76*, 659–665. [CrossRef]
7. Scott, T.W.; Chow, E.; Strickman, D.; Kittayapong, P.; Wirtz, R.A.; Lorenz, L.H.; Edman, J.D. Blood-Feeding Patterns of Aedes aegypti (Diptera: Culicidae) Collected in a Rural Thai Village. *J. Med. Entomol.* **1993**, *30*, 922–927. [CrossRef]
8. Scott, T.W.; Amerasinghe, P.H.; Morrison, A.C.; Lorenz, L.H.; Clark, G.G.; Strickman, D.; Kittayapong, P.; Edman, J.D. Longitudinal Studies of Aedes aegypti (Diptera: Culicidae) in Thailand and Puerto Rico: Blood Feeding Frequency. *J. Med. Entomol.* **2000**, *37*, 89–101. [CrossRef]
9. Maciel-de-Freitas, R.; Marques, W.d.A.; Peres, R.C.; Cunha, S.P.d.; Lourenço-de-Oliveira, R. Variation in *Aedes aegypti* (diptera: culicidae) container productivity in a slum and a suburban district of rio de janeiro during dry and wet seasons. *Memórias Inst. Oswaldo Cruz* **2007**, *102*, 489–496. [CrossRef]
10. Runge-Ranzinger, S.; McCall, P.J.; Kroeger, A.; Horstick, O. Dengue disease surveillance: An updated systematic literature review. *Trop. Med. Int. Health* **2014**, *19*, 1116–1160. [CrossRef]
11. Jourdain, F.; Samy, A.M.; Hamidi, A.; Bouattour, A.; Alten, B.; Faraj, C.; Roiz, D.; Petrić, D.; Pérez-Ramírez, E.; Velo, E.; et al. Towards harmonisation of entomological surveillance in the Mediterranean area. *PLoS Neglected Trop. Dis.* **2019**, *13*, e0007314. [CrossRef] [PubMed]
12. Codeço, C.T.; Lima, A.W.S.; Araújo, S.C.; Lima, J.B.P.; Maciel-de Freitas, R.; Honório, N.A.; Galardo, A.K.R.; Braga, I.A.; Coelho, G.E.; Valle, D. Surveillance of Aedes aegypti: Comparison of House Index with Four Alternative Traps. *PLoS Neglected Trop. Dis.* **2015**, *9*, 1–23. [CrossRef] [PubMed]
13. Leandro, A.; Maciel-de Freitas, R. Development of an Integrated Surveillance System to Improve Preparedness for Arbovirus Outbreaks in a Dengue Endemic Setting: Descriptive Study. *JMIR Public Health Surveill* **2024**, *10*, e62759. [CrossRef] [PubMed]
14. Leandro, A.S.; Chiba de Castro, W.A.; Garey, M.V.; Maciel-de Freitas, R. Spatial analysis of dengue transmission in an endemic city in Brazil reveals high spatial structuring on local dengue transmission dynamics. *Sci. Rep.* **2024**, *14*, 8930. [CrossRef]
15. Leandro, A.; Chiba de Castro, W.; Defante, R.; Delai, R.; Villela, D.; Maciel-de Freitas, R. Citywide Integrated Aedes aegypti Mosquito Surveillance as Early Warning System for Arbovirus Transmission, Brazil. *Emerg. Infect. Dis.* **2022**, *28*, 707. [CrossRef]
16. Leandro, A.d.S.; Ayala, M.J.C.; Lopes, R.D.; Martins, C.A.; Maciel-de Freitas, R.; Villela, D.A.M. Entomo-Virological Aedes aegypti Surveillance Applied for Prediction of Dengue Transmission: A Spatio-Temporal Modeling Study. *Pathogens* **2023**, *12*, 4. [CrossRef]
17. Runge-Ranzinger, S.; Horstick, O.; Marx, M.; Kroeger, A. What does dengue disease surveillance contribute to predicting and detecting outbreaks and describing trends? *Trop. Med. Int. Health* **2008**, *13*, 1022–1041. [CrossRef]
18. Pepin, K.; Leach, C.; Marques-Toledo, C.; Laass, K.; Paixao, K.; Luis, A.; Hayman, D.; Johnson, N.; Buhnerkempe, M.; Carver, S.; et al. Utility of mosquito surveillance data for spatial prioritization of vector control against dengue viruses in three Brazilian cities. *Parasites Vectors* **2015**, *8*, 98. [CrossRef]
19. Leandro, A.; Oliveira, F.; Defante, R.; Rivas, A.; Martins, C.; Silva, I.; Villela, D.; Teixeira, M.; Xavier, S.; Maciel-de Freitas, R. The fuzzy system ensembles entomological, epidemiological, demographic and environmental data to unravel the dengue transmission risk in an endemic city. *BMC Public Health* **2024**, *24*, 2587. [CrossRef]
20. Gurgel-Gonçalves, R.; Oliveira, W.; Croda, J. The greatest Dengue epidemic in Brazil: Surveillance, Prevention, and Control. *Rev. Soc. Bras. Med. Trop.* **2024**, *57*, e002032024. [CrossRef]
21. Lee, K.S.; Lai, Y.L.; Lo, S.; Barkham, T.; Aw, P.; Ooi, P.; Tai, J.; Hibberd, M.; Johansson, P.; Khoo, S.; et al. Dengue Virus Surveillance for Early Warning, Singapore. *Emerg. Infect. Dis.* **2010**, *16*, 847–849. [CrossRef]
22. World Health Organization. *Handbook for Integrated Vector Management*; World Health Organization: Geneva, Switzerland, 2012.
23. Beier, J.; Keating, J.; Githure, J.; Macdonald, M.; Impoinvil, D.; Novak, R. Integrated vector management for malaria control. *Malar. J.* **2008**, *7* (Suppl. S1), S4. [CrossRef] [PubMed]
24. da Silva, L.M.I.; Maciel-de Freitas, R.; Paiva, M.H.S.; da Luz Wallau, G., Horizons of the Future: Preparedness and Response. In *Current Topics in Microbiology and Immunology*; Springer: Berlin/Heidelberg, Germany, 2025; pp. 1–25. [CrossRef]

25. Jose, S.A.; Mathew, K.; Hamna Mariyam, K.B.; Jirawattanapanit, A.; Weraprasertsakun, A. Analyzing and forecasting dengue fever incidence in Thailand: A comprehensive study for public health preparedness. *Int. J. Biomath.* **2024** . [CrossRef]
26. Jose, S.A.; Raja, R.; Omede, B.I.; Agarwal, R.P.; Alzabut, J.; Cao, J.; Balas, V.E. Mathematical modeling on co-infection: Transmission dynamics of Zika virus and Dengue fever. *Nonlinear Dyn.* **2023**, *111*, 4879–4914. [CrossRef]
27. Joseph, D.; Ramachandran, R.; Alzabut, J.; Jose, S.A.; Khan, H. A Fractional-Order Density-Dependent Mathematical Model to Find the Better Strain of Wolbachia. *Symmetry* **2023**, *15*, 845. [CrossRef]
28. Freitas, A.R.R.; Angerami, R.; Zuben, A.; Donalisio, M. Introduction and transmission of Zika virus in Brazil: New challenges for the Americas. *Rev. Inst. Med. Trop. São Paulo* **2016**, *58*, 24. [CrossRef] [PubMed]
29. Barreto, M.; Barral-Netto, M.; Stabeli, R.; Almeida-Filho, N.; Vasconcelos, P.; Teixeira, M.; Buss, P.; Gadelha, P. Zika virus and microcephaly in Brazil: A scientific agenda. *Lancet* **2016**, *387*, 919–921. [CrossRef]
30. Zanluca, C.; De Melo, V.C.A.; Mosimann, A.L.P.; Dos Santos, G.I.V.; dos Santos, C.N.D.; Luz, K. First report of autochthonous transmission of Zika virus in Brazil. *Mem. Inst. Oswaldo Cruz* **2015**, *110*, 569–572. [CrossRef]
31. Faria, N.R.; do Socorro da Silva Azevedo, R.; Kraemer, M.U.G.; Souza, R.; Cunha, M.S.; Hill, S.C.; Thézé, J.; Bonsall, M.B.; Bowden, T.A.; Rissanen, I.; et al. Zika virus in the Americas: Early epidemiological and genetic findings. *Science* **2016**, *352*, 345–349. [CrossRef] [PubMed]
32. Mhamadi, M.; Mencattelli, G.; Gaye, A.; Ndiaye, E.H.; Sow, A.A.; Faye, M.; Ndione, M.H.D.; Diagne, M.M.; Mhamadi, M.; Faye, O.; et al. Rapid On-Site Detection of Arboviruses by a Direct RT-qPCR Assay. *Biosensors* **2023**, *13*, 1035. [CrossRef]
33. Bokobza, L. Near Infrared Spectroscopy. *J. Near Infrared Spectrosc.* **1998**, *6*, 3–17. [CrossRef]
34. Sakudo, A.; Suganuma, Y.; Kobayashi, T.; Onodera, T.; Ikuta, K. Near-infrared spectroscopy: Promising diagnostic tool for viral infections. *Biochem. Biophys. Res. Commun.* **2006**, *341*, 279–284. [CrossRef]
35. Sikulu-Lord, M.; de Freitas, R.M. Application of Infrared Techniques for Characterisation of Vector-Borne Disease Vectors. In *Infrared Spectroscopy*; IntechOpen: London, UK, 2022; Chapter 7. [CrossRef]
36. Fernandes, J.N.; dos Santos, L.M.B.; Chouin-Carneiro, T.; Pavan, M.G.; Garcia, G.A.; David, M.R.; Beier, J.C.; Dowell, F.E.; de Freitas, R.M.; Sikulu-Lord, M.T. Rapid, noninvasive detection of Zika virus in Aedes aegypti mosquitoes by near-infrared spectroscopy. *Sci. Adv. Am. Assoc. Adv. Sci. (AAAS)* **2018**, *4*, eaat0496. [CrossRef]
37. Batistuti Sawazaki, M.R.; Bachour Junior, B.; Mulato, M.; de Oliveira Filho, J.I. Machine Learning-Assisted Infectious Disease Detection in Low-Income Areas: Toward Rapid Triage of Dengue and Zika Virus Using Open-Source Hardware. *Adv. Intell. Discov.* **2025**. [CrossRef]
38. Abu-Mostafa, Y.; Magdon-Ismail, M.; Lin, H.T. *Learning from Data: A Short Course*; AMLBook: Pasadena, CA, USA, 2012.
39. Martinez, A.; Kak, A. PCA versus LDA. *IEEE Trans. Pattern Anal. Mach. Intell.* **2001**, *23*, 228–233. [CrossRef]
40. Teng, C.H.; Hsu, W.H.; Busey, T.; Schneider, B.; Moses, K.; Zheng, W.S.; Lai, J.H.; Yuen, P.; Aleksic, P.; Wagner, M.; et al. LDA (Linear Discriminant Analysis). In *Encyclopedia of Biometrics*; Springer: Berlin/Heidelberg, Germany, 2009; pp. 1–899. [CrossRef]
41. Murphy, K.P. *Machine Learning: A Probabilistic Perspective*; MIT Press: Cambridge, MA, USA, 2013. [CrossRef]
42. Bishop, C.M. *Pattern Recognition and Machine Learning (Information Science and Statistics)*; Springer: Berlin/Heidelberg, Germany, 2006; pp. 1–738. [CrossRef]
43. Cristianini, N.; Shawe-Taylor, J. *An Introduction to Support Vector Machines and Other Kernel-based Learning Methods*; Cambridge University Press: Cambridge, UK, 2000.
44. Boser, B.E.; Guyon, I.M.; Vapnik, V.N. A Training Algorithm for Optimal Margin Classifiers. In Proceedings of the 5th Annual Workshop on Computational Learning Theory (COLT'92), Pittsburgh, PA, USA, 27–29 July 1992; pp. 144–152.
45. Takahashi, A.; Flores, E.A.; Maciel-de-Freitas, R.; Kariyawasam, T.; Sikulu-Lord, M.T. Comparative Evaluation of a Portable and Benchtop Near-Infrared Spectrometers for Characterizing the Age and Blood Feeding History of *Aedes aegypti* Mosquitoes in the Lab. *Preprints* **2025**, 2025081494. [CrossRef]

Tropical Medicine and Infectious Disease

MDPI

Review

An Overview of Dengue Knowledge, Attitudes, and Practices (KAPs) Among the General Public in Sri Lanka: A Review and Meta-Analysis of Questionnaire-Based Surveys from 2000–2023

Nilmini Chandrasena [1,*], Dileepa Ediriweera [2], Deshaka Jayakody [1], Nayana Gunathilaka [1] and Ranjan Premaratna [3]

1 Department of Parasitology, Faculty of Medicine, University of Kelaniya, Ragama 11010, Sri Lanka; djayak.mem2403@pg.kln.ac.lk (D.J.); n.gunathilaka@kln.ac.lk (N.G.)
2 Health Data Science Unit, Faculty of Medicine, University of Kelaniya, Ragama 11010, Sri Lanka; dileepa@kln.ac.lk
3 Department of Medicine, Faculty of Medicine, University of Kelaniya, Ragama 11010, Sri Lanka; ranjanp64@kln.ac.lk
* Correspondence: nilmini@kln.ac.lk

Abstract

The objective was to conduct a review and meta-analysis of questionnaire-based surveys of dengue knowledge, attitudes, perceptions, and practices (KAP)s among the general public in Sri Lanka as no prior island-wide survey existed. The electronic database PubMed and other bibliography were searched for literature on dengue questionnaire-based KAP surveys in Sri Lanka from 2000–2023. Data pertaining to the three domains were extracted from sixteen eligible articles, pooled, and analyzed separately using random effect models. Meta-analyses of the three domains were performed using R version 3.6.3. The population surveyed (8955) was <0.045% of the total Sri Lankan population. The publication frequency increased over time and surveys were distributed in Colombo and suburbs 43.7% (7/16), Kandy 25% (4/16,) Gampaha 12.5% (2/16), and 6.3% (1/16) one each in Kurunegala, Matara, Batticaloa, and Jaffna. Knowledge on dengue transmission, vector breeding, and fever as a symptom was >80%, while on vector species, preferred feeding times, recurrence of dengue it was > 55% and on warning signs of severity it was 25%. Attitudes towards community participation in dengue prevention activities and knowledge of dengue risk factors (avoidance of aspirin and dark colored drinks) were poor, while practice of control measures (removal of water collecting receptacles, roof-gutter management) lacked regularity.

Keywords: dengue; knowledge; attitudes; practices; Sri Lanka

1. Introduction

Dengue fever, a mosquito-borne viral infection, stands as the most widespread and rapidly expanding arboviral infection globally [1]. The illness presents as a spectrum of disease manifestations and is categorized into dengue fever (DF) with or without warning signs and severe dengue which includes Dengue Hemorrhagic Fever (DHF)/Dengue Shock Syndrome (DSS) and severe organ impairment as defined by the World Health Organization (WHO) 2009 [2]. The global incidence of dengue has markedly increased over the past two decades [3]. Currently, over half the global population is at risk in 129 countries, with an estimated 10,000 deaths and 100 million symptomatic infections per year [4]. Thus, dengue is an ever-present threat to human health in tropical and subtropical regions of the world where the mosquito vectors *Aedes aegypti* and *A. albopictus* thrive. Approximately 70% of the global burden of dengue is estimated to be in Asia [3].

Sri Lanka is a tropical island nation (population 22 million) situated in the Indian Ocean comprised of nine administrative provinces and 26 districts. Among the Asian countries with a high dengue burden, Sri Lanka ranks amongst the world's 30 most endemic countries [5]. Following the first serological confirmationof dengue in Sri Lanka in 1962, multiple island-wide outbreaks of DF with cases of severe dengue (DHF, DSS) and deaths occurred [6–9]. The magnitude of dengue epidemics increased from early 2000 onwards, with large epidemics documented in years 2002, 2004 and 2017 [8]. In 2005, the National Dengue Control Unit (NDCU) of the Ministry of Health was established to curb the escalating burden of dengue cases [8]. The NDCU implemented dengue prevention programs at district and national level. Pivotal to the sustainability of dengue control is involvement of the community. Thus, improving public awareness, attitudes, and practices on all aspects of dengue has been the focus of social mobilization programs conducted by the NDCU [8]. Activities include declaration of dengue mosquito control week/s, production and dissemination of dengue information, education, and communication (IEC) material to the public aimed at enhancing or creating awareness on preventive strategies and to promote early health-seeking behavior [8]. The communication for behavioral impact (COMBI) approach was implemented to encourage specified behaviors (removal of breeding sites and early medical attention for fever) to target groups (housewives, school principals and teachers, dengue prevention committees and dengue patients) with key messages comprising weekly inspections and clearance of vector breeding sites in home, school, and work environments, seeking treatment for fevers of over two days from a qualified medical doctor and avoidance of anti-inflammatory drugs [8]. These promotional activities mostly happen periodically in anticipation of or during an outbreak of dengue. The impact of these societal interventions has been studied in Sri Lanka via questionnaire-based surveys on KAPs targeting specified communities or subpopulations who were perceived as high-risk groups (school children) or were important in implementation of control strategies (housewives, school teachers, and youth organizations). However, an island-wide survey or a review of dengue KAPs has not reported to date. Thus, the objective was to conduct a review of the literature on questionnaire-based dengue KAP surveys in Sri Lanka with meta-analysis of the three domains.

2. Materials and Methods

2.1. Search Strategy

A search of the PubMed database was conducted on the 28 December 2023 to identify relevant literature from year 2000 onwards using relevant Medical Subject Headings (MeSH) terms "Dengue/epidemiology", "Dengue/prevention & control", "Sri Lanka", and variations of "Knowledge, Attitudes, and Practices." Additional search techniques were employed to broaden the search. These techniques included searching within titles and abstracts, incorporating alternative keywords and phrases, and exploring related articles and citations. The search was expanded to include terms such as "survey", "questionnaire", "prevention", and "treatment" within titles and abstracts. We also used wildcards and truncation to capture variations of terms, ensuring that our search was not restricted by specific wording. The titles and abstracts of the search output were screened independently by two investigators (Nilmini Chandrasena and Nayana Gunathilake) for relevance and eligibility based on inclusion criteria. In the event of controversy, a third investigator (Ranjan Premaratna) was consulted.

2.2. Inclusion Criteria

The inclusion criteria comprised of cross-sectional studies with quantitative data on dengue-related KAPs were conducted in Sri Lanka and utilized questionnaire-based methodologies. The titles and abstracts of the articles were screened by three authors and those not meeting the inclusion criteria were excluded.

2.3. Data Extraction for Analysis

Two investigators (Deshaka Jayakody and Nilmini Chandrasena) performed data extraction in which DJ extracted data into a pre-formed data extraction template while NC cross-checked the extracted data. The data extracted were the reported outcomes of survey questions addressing any of the KAP domains per study. Outcomes reported as percentages were converted to numbers where necessary. Survey items across studies were categorized under the three domains. The items under the knowledge domain included knowledge on viral etiology, transmission, vector bionomics, symptoms of infection, warning signs of severity, re-infection events, preventive, and management measures (hydration, avoidance of aspirin and dark colored drinks or food). Items under the attitudes domain included perceptions of severity, treatability, preventability, treatment-seeking behaviors, support for premise inspection, and participation in community clean-up activities. The items under the practices domain included practice of individual protection measures (mosquito nets, repellants) and activities pertaining to prevention of mosquito breeding (environmental clean-up, covering water-holding containers, clearance of roof gutters). A table was created to organize data, accounting for variability in study tools and surveyed items.

2.4. Meta-Analysis of Data in the Three Domains

There were differences in the number of questions in the surveys. We, therefore, considered each question as a separate outcome and conducted the analysis. To assess the collective outcome of each question within KAP surveys, we conducted a separate meta-analysis. Heterogeneity between studies was evaluated using the I^2 statistic and the Cochran Q test. A random-effects meta-analysis of proportions was conducted to calculate pooled estimates, accounting for heterogeneity [10]. Inverse variance weighting and the DerSimonian–Laird method were used to pool the estimates [11]. Statistical analyses were performed (Dileepa Ediriweera) using R version 3.6.3. The "meta" package was used for meta-analyses of proportions. The "dmetar" package was used to identify outliers and influential studies.

3. Results

A total of 93 articles were obtained from the PubMed search using MeSH terms. Additionally, 11 more articles were found through bibliography and Google Scholar searches, adding up to a total of 105 articles. Of these, 88 were excluded, as these were determined to be irrelevant to KAP studies and/or Sri Lanka. Ultimately, a total of 16 articles were included in the review (Figure 1).

Questionnaire-based KAP surveys on dengue were published from 2012 onwards in Sri Lanka with only five surveys being reported during the first six years of scrutiny (2012–2017) compared to eleven studies being documented over the subsequent six years (2018–2023). The majority of the studies were conducted in urban and semi-urban areas in the districts of Colombo and suburbs 43.7% (7/16,) Kandy 25% (4/16), and Gampaha 12.5% (2/16), while the districts of Kurunegala, Matara, Batticaloa, and Jaffna reported a single study each. The population screened for dengue KAPs in Sri Lanka was a minority (0.045% n = 8955). Specified populations were mostly targeted such as community members residing in high-endemic areas (seven studies, n = 4667), high-risk populations such as school children (two studies, n = 2331), undergraduates (single study, n = 384), hospital-based studies on patients receiving indoor care for dengue (two studies, n = 332) outpatients (single study, n = 500), parents of children hospitalized for fever (single study, n = 86) and subpopulations involved in implementing control, such as housewives (single study, n = 400), school teachers (single study, n = 105), urban youths (single study, n = 150), (Table 1).

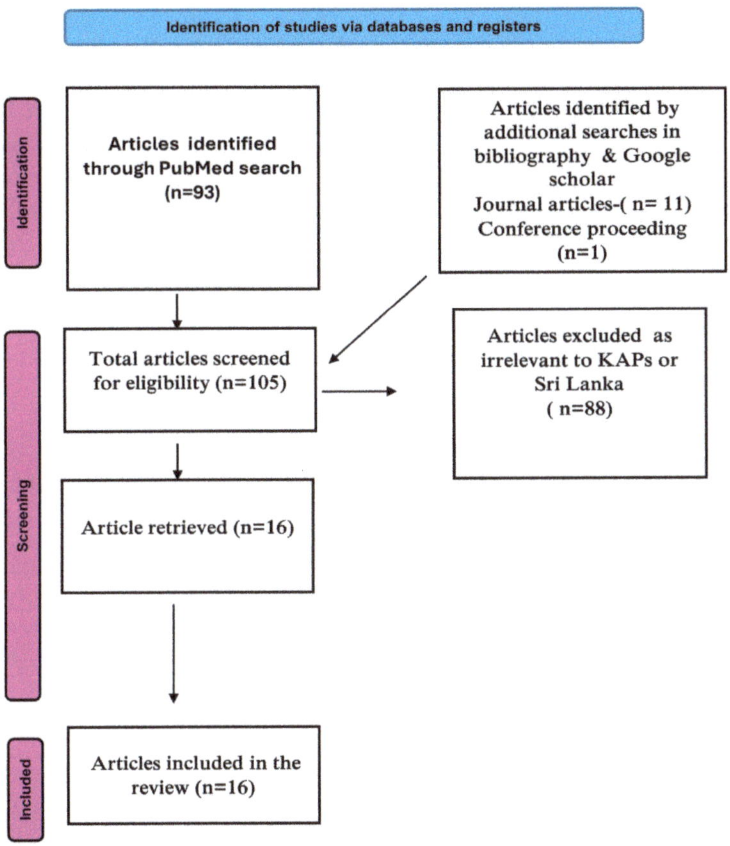

Figure 1. Flowchart of papers included in the review.

Table 1. Publications included in the review on dengue knowledge, attitudes, and practices surveys in Sri Lanka.

Author	Article Title	Year	Region of Sri Lanka	Sample Size	Age Group	Study Population	Main Outcomes of the Study
Chanyasanha et al. [12]	Factors influencing preventive behaviors for dengue infection among housewives in Colombo, Sri Lanka	2015	Colombo municipality	400	20+	Housewives	69.2% had dengue knowledge 91.5% positive attitudes 58.5% preventive knowledge
Disanayaka et al. [13]	Knowledge, attitudes, and practices (KAP) about dengue prevention among residents in Ratmalana medical officer of health area	2017	Attidiya North	312	18+	Community members (Ratmalana MOH area)	>90% had dengue knowledge >90% positive attitudes to early medical attention and source reduction 65% participation in environmental clean ups

Table 1. *Cont.*

Author	Article Title	Year	Region of Sri Lanka	Sample Size	Age Group	Study Population	Main Outcomes of the Study
Gayathri et al. [14]	Knowledge, attitudes, and practices towards dengue among undergraduate students at a University in Sri Lanka	2021	University of Peradeniya	384	20–30	Undergraduate students	40–60% in health-related faculties had satisfactory knowledge <20% in non-health-related faculties had satisfactory knowledge Overall, 60.9% had fair-satisfactory practice scores
Gunadhasam et al. [15]	Knowledge, attitudes, and practices on dengue prevention among secondary school students in university community project area	2021	Batticaloa District	137	14–16	Secondary school students	68.6% had good knowledge 67.9% had good practices 44.5% had poor attitudes
Gunasekara et al. [16]	Knowledge, attitudes, and practices regarding dengue fever in a suburban community in Sri Lanka	2012	Colombo district	349	<20–55+	Community members (Boralesgamuwa MOH area)	58% had satisfactory knowledge score (>70) 37% had satisfactory attitudes (score > 75) 85% had good practices; (score > 70)
Jayalath et al. [17]	Knowledge and attitudes regarding dengue fever among the outdoor patients of the teaching hospital Peradeniya, Sri Lanka	2018	Teaching hospital Peradeniya	500	20–70	Outpatients at Teaching Hospital Peradeniya	46.5% had >average knowledge
Jayawickreme et al. [18]	A study on knowledge, attitudes, and practices regarding dengue fever, its prevention and management among dengue patients presenting to a tertiary care hospital in Sri Lanka	2021	Colombo	132	13+	Dengue patients at SJH	62% had dengue prevention awareness 51% had dengue management awareness
Kumanan et al. [19]	A study on knowledge, attitudes, and practices regarding dengue among hospitalized patients from Northern Sri Lanka	2018	Jaffna	200	12+	Dengue patients at Teaching Hospital Jaffna	>90%–had early health-seeking behavior, Prevention, mostly avoidance of mosquito bites, with low focus on source reduction
Nazeer et al. [20]	Awareness of dengue fever among the urban youth in Colombo and its Suburbs, Sri Lanka in November 2014	2015	Colombo and suburbs	150	16–25	Urban youth	48% knew dengue specific features Awareness on substances to avoid during illness; 66% NSAIDS 16% unspecified food items 32% believed in papaya leaf extract therapy
Pavithra et al. [21]	Awareness, attitudes, and preventive measures practiced towards dengue fever by the teachers of three schools in Colombo District	2015	Colombo District	105	20–60	Teachers in the Colombo District	20% had good knowledge 68% had fair knowledge 12% poor knowledge 65% regarded prevention a self-responsibility
Perera et al. [22]	Household-based survey on knowledge, attitudes, and practices towards dengue infection and prevention in a semi-urban area (Ja-Ela MOH Area)	2021	Gampaha District	510	18+	Ja-Ela MOH Area	Good awareness; 56.5%, Good attitudes; 52.9%, Good practices; 50.7%
Radhika et al. [23]	Level of awareness of dengue disease among school children in Gampaha District, Sri Lanka, and effect of school-based health education programs on improving knowledge and practices	2019	Gampaha District	2194	13–15	School children	Knowledge prior to health education (HE) Good; 46.3% Excellent; 3% After HE 41.8% had excellent knowledge

Table 1. *Cont.*

Author	Article Title	Year	Region of Sri Lanka	Sample Size	Age Group	Study Population	Main Outcomes of the Study
Rajapaksha et al. [24]	health-seeking behaviors, dengue prevention behaviors and community capacity for sustainable dengue prevention in a highly dengue-endemic area, Sri Lanka	2023	Kurunegala District	496	18–70	Community in a high-endemic region	Preventive behaviors; 19.2% Early medical attention; 44.6%
Udaynga et al. [25]	Comprehensive evaluation of demographic, socio-economic and other associated risk factors affecting the occurrence of dengue incidence among Colombo and Kandy Districts of Sri Lanka: a cross-sectional study	2018	Colombo and Kandy	2000	0–55+	Community in high dengue incidence regions	dengue affected groups (test) had better knowledge on illness, than dengue-non-affected (control)
Udayanga et al. [26]	Socio-economic, knowledge, attitudes, and practices (KAP), household related and demographic based appearance of non-dengue infected individuals in high dengue risk areas of Kandy District, Sri Lanka	2018	Kandy District	1000	15–55+	Non-infected individuals in high-risk regions	Dengue knowledge; good-medium except in Kundasale and Kandy municipality Good preventive measures and high environmental cleanliness
Wickremasinghe et al. [27]	Knowledge, attitudes, and practices of a selected group of parents on pre-hospital management of fever in children in a dengue-endemic area of Southern Sri Lanka	2021	Teaching Hospital Karapitiya and District General Hospital, Matara	86	20–40+	Parents of children with fever hospitalized at Teaching Hospital Karapitiya and District General Hospital, Matara	Dengue risk awareness 27.9%, 55.8 knew NSAIDs were best avoided but 32.56 preferred NSAIDs for fever management 89.53% knew hydration was important

3.1. Study Tool Validity and Reliability

The study tools utilized were validated and pre-tested in three studies [12,14,22], only pre-tested in five [13,16,23,28,29], and only validated in four [18,19,24,30] studies. Two studies reported the reliability of the study tool by calculating the Cronbach's α coefficients with scores ranging from 0.83–0.98 [12,24]. The questionnaires were self-administered (n = 8) or interviewer-administered (n = 7) while one was administered online via a social media-network.

3.2. Knowledge Domain

Meta-analysis of the knowledge domain indicates that the Sri Lankan population in urban and suburban areas had good (≥80%) knowledge on transmission aspects of dengue [13,16,17,19,21,22,25,26], vector bionomics which included breeding preferences [14,16–18,20,23,25,26] the day-biting nature of vectors [15–19,22,26], and viral etiology [14,26]. The knowledge of mosquito vector species was 55% [13,16,17,19–22,25,26], but the vector adaptations to breed in brackish and polluted water were limited [13,14]. Knowledge of dengue as a febrile infection was good (>80%) [13–17,19–22,26]. However, knowledge of other symptoms (abdominal pain, rash,) or severity indicators such as low-urine output and bleeding manifestations was low (25%) (Table 2).

Knowledge of the potential for recurrence of dengue due to multiple viral serotypes [13,17–19,26] and association of outbreaks with rainy season was >60% [14–16,22]. Less than half (41%) were aware that there was no specific medicine to cure dengue [15,18,20]. The awareness of dengue risks was surprisingly low (27.9%) in some high-endemic residential environments [25,27]. Factors affecting the knowledge domain were level of education [12,13,17–19,22], family income [12,17,22], and past dengue experience [22,25]. Media (television and radio broad casts) were preferred sources of information [13,16,19], while newspapers, schools, and health personnel also contributed [13,16,19] (Table 2).

Table 2. Meta-analysis of the knowledge domain in dengue KAP surveys (2000–2023) in Sri Lanka.

Dengue Transmission Knowledge	No. Studies	Total Sample Size	Correct Responses	I^2	Random-Effects Model (95% CI)
Dengue is mosquito-borne	8	7255	6324	99.8%	87.3% [64–99.4%]
Vector species	7	5991	4322	99.4%	55.0% [34.7–74.5%]
Biting times of vector	7	5828	3647	98.5%	66.4% [52.8–78.8%]
Vector breeding characteristics	8	6128	5690	97.8%	88.8% [81.1–94.7%]
Disease knowledge					
Viral etiology	2	4384	3768	0%	86% [84.9–87%]
Serotypes	1	4000	2468	NA	61.7% [60.2–63.2%]
Febrile infection	8	6141	5514	99.7%	80.1% [53.1–97.2%]
Other dengue symptoms	2	462	98	98.9%	25.4% [0.3–70.%]
Recurrence of dengue	5	5144	3850	97.5%	0.68.4% [56.1–79.4%]
No specific medicine	3	419	180	97.4%	41.5% [15.4–70.4%]
Papaya leaf extract does not cure	2	282	113	78.6%	39.7% [27.7–52.3%]
Association with rainy season	4	1380	794	99.5%	65% [28.5–93.5%]

3.3. Attitudes Domain

Attitudes towards perceived dengue severity with potential for fatality [15,17–19], susceptibility regardless of age [13], treatability [13,17], preventability [19], early treatment-seeking behavior from qualified medical practitioners [13,14,17,20–22,24], support for premise inspection and fogging [15,22,26] were positive (>75%) (Table 3). Attitudes towards maintaining hydration during illness [13,14,19,21,22] were average (>55%). Only a minority had positive attitudes towards Ayurveda (5%), while beliefs on papaya leaf extracts to cure dengue had more acceptability (32% were strongly positive and 22% were positive) [17,20]. Negative attitudes were reported with regard to the perceived onus of dengue control activities, with 73.6% perceiving it as the government's responsibility [12,22], 35% perceiving it as individual's responsibility [14], and 58% perceiving it a shared responsibility between the state and individuals [17,22] (Table 3). Factors having a positive impact on attitudes domain were high family income, male gender, past dengue experience, employment status, and health awareness programs tailored for specific demographic groups [12,22–24].

Table 3. Meta-analysis of the domain of attitudes in dengue KAP surveys (2000–2023) in Sri Lanka.

Illness Perceptions/Management	No. Studies	Total Sample Size	Correct Responses	I^2	Random-Effects Model (95% CI)
Dengue fatality	4	969	833	97.5%	83.1% [64.3–95.9%]
Preventable	1	200	152	NA	76.% [69.5–81.7%]
Susceptibility regardless of age	1	312	305	NA	97.8% [95.43–99.1%]
Treatable	2	812	758	93.7%	94.5% [86.4–99.2%]
Early treatment from a medical practitioner	7	2472	1929	98.4%	82.4% [68.7–92.9%]
Ayurveda as initial treatment	1	500	26	NA	5.2% [3.4–7.5%]
Hydration/oral fluids	5	1102	615	99%	56% [25.9–83.9%]
Control is the government's responsibility	2	894	558	99.8%	73.6% [6.8–100.%]
Control is a self-responsibility	1	120	42	NA	35.% [26.5–44.2%]
Control is both individual and state responsibility	2	1010	584	96.3%	58.% [41.9–73.3%]
Support for premise inspection and/fogging	3	1647	1226	79.9%	75.3% [69.7–80.%]

3.4. Practices Domain

The practice of mosquito source reduction measures such as clearance of water collecting receptacles outdoors [15,16,18,21,24], covering water tanks, wells and containers [12,15], and cleaning and scrubbing outdoor water-holding containers [15–17,19,21,22,24,26] was good (>70%), but management of indoor breeding sites was barely adequate (<60%) [13,22,24] (Table 4). The management of roof gutters was less than adequate (44.5%) [17,24]. Personal protection methods were practiced by <55%; these include the use of mosquito nets 45.7% [15,17], mosquito coils 43.8% [15,17,19,26], repellants 19.3% [17,19] insecticides 27% [17,19,22] and protective clothing 54.7% [15] (Table 4).

Table 4. Meta-analysis of the practices domain in dengue KAP surveys (2000-2023) in Sri Lanka.

Preventive Practices	No. Studies	Total Sample	Correct Responses	I^2	Random-Effects Model (95% CI)
Scrubbing water containers	8	3312	2483	99.3%	72.4% [52.5–88.6%]
Remove water in outdoor receptacles	5	1234	1041	87.1%	86% [79.7–91.3%]
Remove water in indoor receptacles	3	1318	776	99.3%	58.3% [26.0–87%]
Roof-gutter management	2	996	444	95.3%	44.5% [30.7–58.8%]
Cover wells and tanks	2	537	478	0.0%	89.1% [86.3–91.6%]
Use mosquito nets	4	5100	2286	85.3%	45.7% [40.5–51%]
Protective clothing	1	137	75	NA	54.74 [46–63.3%]
Mosquito coils	3	4700	2930	99.4%	43.8% [16.9–72.8%]
Insecticides	3	1210	364	93.0%	27% [17.8–37.3%]
Repellant use	2	700	212	99.2%	19.3% [0- 63.2%]
Physical rest	2	696	492	94.6%	71.7% [56.3–84.9%]
Paracetamol as antipyretic	3	896	499	89.3%	57.3% [47.2–67.2%]
Avoid NSAIDs	2	849	269	96.8%	32.9% [16.6–51.7%]
Avoid dark colored drinks	3	981	267	99.5%	37.1% [2.6–82.8%]

Except for physical rest implemented by 71.1% [13,14], other practices related to home-based care of dengue patients were barely adequate (<60%); paracetamol for fever management was 57.3% [13,14,19], avoidance of non-steroidal anti-inflammatory drugs (NSAID)s was 32.9% [16,17], and avoidance of dark colored drinks was 37.1% [13,17,18] (Table 4). Factors influencing positive practices were age (25–30 years), dengue knowledge, positive attitudes, family income, unemployment (practices were better among the unemployed), and past dengue experience [12,22] (Table 4).

4. Discussion

This review provides an overview of dengue KAP studies conducted in Sri Lanka from 2000–2023. Although the number of studies included in this review was low, this review is the first to report an overall assessment of dengue KAPs in Sri Lanka. On comparison with dengue KAP reviews in the region, the number of studies in Sri Lanka was similar in range to that of Philippines but low compared to Malaysia and high compared to Thailand [28–30]. The population screened was just a minority.

Meta-analysis of the knowledge domain indicates that the Sri Lankan population in urban and suburban areas had good (≥80%) knowledge on transmission dynamics and viral etiology and febrile nature of dengue infection. (see Table 2). These knowledge rates were much higher than those reported for the Southeast Asian region [31]. Awareness of basic illness features of dengue in Sri Lanka (flue-like illness) was consistent with studies in the region (Philippines, Laos) [28,32]. The low knowledge (25%) on severity indicators such as rash, abdominal pain, and bleeding manifestations was similar to a report in Laos where most (>70%) knew that dengue caused fever but only 18.2% knew of rash, and 3% of bleeding tendencies [32].

The knowledge gaps on warning signs could lead to delayed hospitalization and fatalities. Good public knowledge on dengue transmission may be attributed to the consistent efforts of the Ministry of Health and NDCU to educate the general public on dengue prevention during or prior to outbreaks. The high literacy rates (males, 93.63% and females, 91.3%) particularly in the urban and suburban settings perhaps play a role in the assimilation of the core health messages. These findings are consistent with studies reported in Vietnam, Malaysia, and Tamil Nadu [33–35]. In contrast, in the Philippines, the level of education was inversely associated with dengue knowledge [28].

Health education is an important component of dengue control as a correlation with increased mortality and low dengue knowledge has been documented [30]. Deficiencies noted on home-management aspects such as avoidance of NSAIDS and dark colored drinks and foods such as coke, coffee, and chocolate require more focus in awareness programs. Therefore, developing a national communication strategy that is consistent and timely to build long-term national awareness is suggested. Positive attitudes towards dengue severity perceptions and management in Sri Lanka were similar to those reported in Vietnam, Nepal, and Yemen [33,36,37]. Seeking early medical assistance (Western medicine) was comparable to Philippines, Vietnam, and Tamil Nadu [28,33,35]. In contrast, a study in Malaysia reported that only 50.8% would seek medical assistance if a child with dengue was restless or lethargic [29].

Despite the low faith in Ayurvedic treatment, positive beliefs on papaya leaf extracts were reported. Complimentary substances such as papaya leaf extracts with reported platelet-increasing properties were highly used in Malaysia and the Philippines [29,38]. The negative attitude towards dengue control responsibilities in Sri Lanka was similarly reported in the Philippines, Vietnam, and Tamil Nadu [28,33,35]. However, attitudes towards supporting premise inspection and fogging were positive (>75%) in Sri Lanka. Conduction of awareness programs in schools and other educational institutes on a regular basis may be an option for instilling a sense of community responsibility and thereby improve attitudes among the younger generations [23]. The value of school-based health education programs for dengue control has been widely reported in the literature [39,40].

The practice of source reduction measures was mostly limited to house and garden premises and lacked regularity [13,16]. Public areas such as roads, sidewalks, and neighboring premises were not attended due to time constraints and or fear of disrupting public relations. Attention to water collecting receptacles indoors (58.3%) and management of roof gutters (44.5%) was less than adequate. Regional disparities were noted in application of preventive practices with certain regions focusing more on individual protection methods, or source reduction while some practiced both [12,13,16,19,25]. Public satisfaction was reportedly low regarding the state control efforts [20,21]. Instead of penalizing the public for not clearing vector breeding sites in their properties, a more community-friendly approach by the local authorities is suggested, particularly in clean-up of state-owned public places. Regular removal of solid waste (weekly or biweekly) by the municipality is mandatory to maintain environments free of clutter. The COMBI approach needs to be reinforced and strengthened to motivate the public to change their risk-behaviors.

5. Limitations

The study outcomes may not be representative of dengue KAPs in the general population of Sri Lanka as most surveys targeted specific populations. The variations of the study tools (questionnaires) may have affected the outcome of the review while the comprehensiveness of the literature search may have been limited by the selectivity of MESH terms used in the search. The responses in the domains of attitudes and practices may have been influenced by social desirable bias. Temporal changes on knowledge and behaviors patterns were not analyzed as targeted populations differed.

6. Conclusions

Knowledge on dengue transmission and basic illness features among the general public of Sri Lanka was good, but there were notable gaps in the knowledge domain on dengue severity indicators and risk factors. Negative attitudes towards dengue control responsibilities, deficiencies in home-based care practices, and irregularity in removal of breeding sites (source reduction practices) were the gaps identified in attitudes and practices domains. Geographic disparities in KAP surveys suggest less focus on peripheral districts that are now reporting dengue cases. These geographic gaps need to be addressed by policymakers and researchers in the future. Concerted efforts are required to bridge the identified gaps. The need for a national communication strategy on dengue that is consistent and timely to build long-term national awareness, a dedicated communication expert, community-capacity building programs for provision of technical skills in maintenance of environments is recommended. Reinforcing the COMBI approach to motivate the public to change their risk-behaviors and the integration of dengue control with other vector-borne disease control programs are suggested for cost-efficacy.

Author Contributions: Conceptualization, N.C., N.G. and R.P. Screening the search output for relevance, N.C., N.G. and R.P. Data extraction and compilation D.J. and N.C. Formal analysis D.E. Writing—original draft N.C. and D.E. Writing—review and editing D.J., R.P. and N.G. No funding was received for this project. All authors have read and agreed to the published version of the manuscript.

Funding: This research received no external funding.

Institutional Review Board Statement: Ethics approval for the study was granted by the Ethics review committee of the Faculty of Medicine, University of Kelaniya, Sri Lanka (Ref. No. P/06/01/2024 approved on 9 April 2024).

Informed Consent Statement: Not applicable.

Data Availability Statement: All relevant data generated and analyzed in the current study are included in the manuscript.

Acknowledgments: The authors gratefully acknowledge the support provided by Chitra M Abeygunasekara, former senior assistant librarian of the Faculty of Medicine, University of Kelaniya, in carrying out the literature search.

Conflicts of Interest: The authors declare no conflicts of interests.

Abbreviations

WHO	World Health Organization
DF	Dengue fever
DHF	Dengue haemrrhagic fever
DSS	Dengue shock syndrome
NDCU	National dengue control unit
IEC	Information, education, and communication
COMBI	Communication for behavioral impact
KAP	Knowledge, attitudes, and practices
MeSH	Medical subject headings
NSAID	Non-steroidal anti-inflammatory drug

References

1. Stanaway, J.D.; Shepard, D.S.; Undurraga, E.A.; Halasa, Y.A.; Coffeng, L.E.; Brady, O.J.; Hay, S.I.; Bedi, N.; Bensenor, I.M.; Castañeda-Orjuela, C.A.; et al. The Global Burden of Dengue: An Analysis from the Global Burden of Disease Study 2013. *Lancet Infect. Dis.* **2016**, *16*, 712–723. [CrossRef] [PubMed]
2. Rezeki Hadinegoro, S.S. Paediatrics and International Child Health The Revised WHO Dengue Case Classification: Does the System Need to Be Modified? The Revised WHO Dengue Case Classification: Does the System Need to Be Modified? *Int. Child Health* **2012**, *32*, 33–38. [CrossRef] [PubMed]
3. Dengue and Severe Dengue. Available online: https://www.who.int/news-room/fact-sheets/detail/dengue-and-severe-dengue (accessed on 20 December 2024).
4. Messina, J.P.; Brady, O.J.; Golding, N.; Kraemer, M.U.G.; Wint, G.R.W.; Ray, S.E.; Pigott, D.M.; Shearer, F.M.; Johnson, K.; Earl, L.; et al. The Current and Future Global Distribution and Population at Risk of Dengue. *Nat. Microbiol.* **2019**, *4*, 1508–1515. [CrossRef]
5. Dengue—Global Situation. Available online: https://www.who.int/emergencies/disease-outbreak-news/item/2023-DON498 (accessed on 20 December 2024).

6. Vitarana, T.; Jayakuru, W.S.; Withane, N. Historical Account of Dengue Haemorrhagic Fever in Sri Lanka. *Dengue Bull.* **1997**, *21*, 117.
7. Messer, W.B.; Vitarana, U.T.; Sivananthan, K.; Elvtigala, J.; Preethimala, L.D.; Ramesh, R.; Withana, N.; Gubler, D.J.; De Silva, A.M. Epidemiology of Dengue in Sri Lanka before and after the Emergence of Epidemic Dengue Hemorrhagic Fever. *Am. J. Trop. Med. Hyg.* **2002**, *66*, 765–773. [CrossRef]
8. NDCU—Sri Lanka Situation. Available online: https://www.dengue.health.gov.lk/web/index.php/en/information/sri-lanka-situation (accessed on 19 May 2025).
9. Tissera, H.A.; Jayamanne, B.D.W.; Raut, R.; Janaki, S.M.D.; Tozan, Y.; Samaraweera, P.C.; Liyanage, P.; Ghouse, A.; Rodrigo, C.; de Silva, A.M.; et al. Severe Dengue Epidemic, Sri Lanka, 2017. *Emerg. Infect. Dis.* **2020**, *26*, 682. [CrossRef]
10. DerSimonian, R.; Laird, N. Meta-Analysis in Clinical Trials. *Control Clin. Trials* **1986**, *7*, 177–188. [CrossRef]
11. Deeks, J.J.; Higgins, J.P.T.; Altman, D.G. Chapter 10: Analysing Data and Undertaking Meta-Analyses. In *Cochrane Handbook for Systematic Reviews of Interventions*; Version 6.3 (Updated February 2022); Higgins, J.P.T., Thomas, J., Chandler, J., Cumpston, M., Li, T., Page, M.J., Welch, V.A., Eds.; Cochrane: London, UK, 2022. Available online: https://training.cochrane.org/handbook/archive/v6.3/chapter-10 (accessed on 19 May 2025).
12. Chanyasanha, C.; Guruge, G.R.; Sujirarat, D. Factors Influencing Preventive Behaviors for Dengue Infection Among Housewives in Colombo, Sri Lanka. *Asia Pac. J. Public Health* **2015**, *27*, 96–104. [CrossRef]
13. Disanayaka, K.M.S.D.K.; Kanchana, K.A.N.G.; Nayanajith, E.G.A.P.; Samarasinghe, K.P.D.B.; Priyangika, K.G.G.; Navaratne, P.B.V. Knowledge, Attitudes and Practices (KAP) About Dengue Prevention Among Residents in Ratmalana Medical Officer of Health Area. 2017. Available online: http://ir.kdu.ac.lk/handle/345/1632 (accessed on 25 May 2025).
14. Gayathri, N.G.N.; Sirisena, P.D.N.N.; Senaratne, U.T.N.; Noordeen, F. Knowledge, Attitude and Practices towards Dengue among Undergraduate Students at a University in Sri Lanka. *Sri Lankan J. Infect. Dis.* **2021**, *11*, 73. [CrossRef]
15. Gunadhasam, S.; Rathnayake, M.L.; Bandara, H.L.; Kartheepan, K.; Sundaresan, K.T. Knowledge, Attitude and Practice on Dengue Prevention among Secondary School Students in University Community Project Area. Annual Student Research Sessions (ASRS-FHCS) 2021/07. 28–31. Available online: https://fhcs.esn.ac.lk/asrs2021 (accessed on 25 May 2025).
16. Gunasekara, T.D.; Velathanthiri, V.G.; Fernando, S.S. Knowledge, Attitudes and Practices Regarding Dengue Fever in a Sub-Urban Community in Sri Lanka. *Galle Med. J.* **2012**, *17*, 10–16. [CrossRef]
17. Jayalath, T.; Ralapanawa, U.; Pathirage, M. Knowledge and Attitude Regarding Dengue Fever among the Outdoor Patients of the Teaching Hospital Peradeniya, Sri Lanka. *Int. J. Med. Res. Health Sci.* **2018**, *7*, 77–84.
18. Jayawickreme, K.P.; Jayaweera, D.K.; Weerasinghe, S.; Warapitiya, D.; Subasinghe, S. A Study on Knowledge, Attitudes and Practices Regarding Dengue Fever, Its Prevention and Management among Dengue Patients Presenting to a Tertiary Care Hospital in Sri Lanka. *BMC Infect. Dis.* **2021**, *21*, 981. [CrossRef] [PubMed]
19. Kumanan, T.; Logeswaran, D. A Study on Knowledge, Attitude and Practices Regarding Dengue among Hospitalized Patients from Northern Sri Lanka. *Sri Lankan J. Infect. Dis.* **2018**, *8*, 127–132. [CrossRef]
20. Nazeer, A.A.A.; de Silva, T.D. Awareness of Dengue Fever among the Urban Youth in Colombo and Its Suburbs, Sri Lanka in November 2014. *GSTF Int. J. Nurs. Heal. Care (JNHC)* **2015**, *3*, 25–29.
21. Pavithra, M.; Opatha, V.; Palliyaguruge, R.; Dissanayake, W. Awareness, Attitude and Preventive Measures Practiced towards Dengue Fever by the Teachers of Three Schools in Colombo District. In Proceedings of the 8th International Research Conference—KDU, in Medicine, Dehiwala-Mount Lavinia, Sri Lanka, 27–28 August 2015; pp. 47–54.
22. Perera, W.L.S.; Perera, P.K.; Wijesundara, C.; Ambagahawita, A.M.; Fernando, S.U.; Udara, S.; Bandaranayaka, K.O. Household-Based Survey on Knowledge, Attitudes, and Practices towards Dengue Infection and Prevention in a Semi-Urban Area (Ja-Ela MOH Area). *Int. J. Med. Parasit. Epidemiol. Sci.* **2021**, *2*, 83–90. [CrossRef]
23. Radhika, N.M.L.; Gunathilaka, N.; Udayanga, L.; Kasturiratne, A.; Abeyewickreme, W. Level of Awareness of Dengue Disease among School Children in Gampaha District, Sri Lanka, and Effect of School-Based Health Education Programmes on Improving Knowledge and Practices. *Biomed. Res. Int.* **2019**, *2019*, 3092073. [CrossRef]
24. Rajapaksha, R.M.N.U.; Abeysena, C.; Balasuriya, A. Health Seeking Behaviours, Dengue Prevention Behaviours and Community Capacity for Sustainable Dengue Prevention in a Highly Dengue Endemic Area, Sri Lanka. *BMC Public Health* **2023**, *23*, 507. [CrossRef]
25. Udayanga, L.; Gunathilaka, N.; Iqbal, M.C.M.; Lakmal, K.; Amarasinghe, U.S.; Abeyewickreme, W. Comprehensive evaluation of demographic, socio-economic and other associated risk factors affecting the occurrence of dengue incidence among Colombo and Kandy Districts of Sri Lanka: A cross-sectional study. *Parasit. Vectors* **2018**, *11*, 478. [CrossRef]
26. Udayanga, L.; Gunathilaka, N.; Iqbal, M.C.M.; Pahalagedara, K.; Amarasinghe, U.S.; Abeyewickreme, W. Socio-Economic, Knowledge Attitude Practices (KAP), Household Related and Demographic Based Appearance of Non-Dengue Infected Individuals in High Dengue Risk Areas of Kandy District, Sri Lanka. *BMC Infect. Dis.* **2018**, *18*, 88. [CrossRef]

27. Wickremasinghe, I.K.; Basnayake, A.N.; Kumara, D.S.; Arachchi, D.K. Knowledge, Attitudes and Practices of a Selected Group of Parents on Pre-Hospital Management of Fever in Children in a Dengue-Endemic Area of Southern Sri Lanka. *Galle Med. J.* **2021**, *26*, 17–22. [CrossRef]
28. Mac Guad, R.; Carandang, R.R.; Solidum, J.N.; Taylor-Robinson, A.W.; Wu, Y.S.; Aung, Y.N.; Low, W.Y.; Sim, M.S.; Sekaran, S.D.; Azizan, N. Different Domains of Dengue Research in the Philippines: A Systematic Review and Meta-Analysis of Questionnaire-Based Studies. *PLoS ONE* **2021**, *16*, e0261412. [CrossRef]
29. Mac Guad, R.; Wu, Y.S.; Aung, Y.N.; Sekaran, S.D.; Wilke, A.B.B.; Low, W.Y.; Sim, M.S.; Carandang, R.R.; Jeffree, M.S.; Taherdoost, H.; et al. Different Domains of Dengue Research in Malaysia: A Systematic Review and Meta-Analysis of Questionnaire-Based Studies. *Int. J. Med. Res. Health Sci.* **2021**, *18*, 4474. [CrossRef]
30. Crowley, J.; Liu, B.; Jan, H. Assessing the Knowledge, Attitudes, and Practices (KAP) of Dengue Fever in Thailand: A Systematic Review and Meta-Analysis. *medRxiv* **2024**. medRxiv:2024.05.04.24306876. [CrossRef]
31. Sotoodeh, J.A.; Mohammad, J.; Arman, A.; Nader, S.; Tahere, A.; Vahid, R. Global systematic review and meta- analysis of knowledge, attitudes, and practices towards dengue fever among the general population. *Asian Pac. J. Trop. Med.* **2024**, *17*, 191–207. [CrossRef]
32. Nalongsack, S.; Yoshida, Y.; Morita, S.; Sosouphanh, K.; Sakamoto, J. Knowledge, attitude and practice regarding dengue among people in Pakse, Laos. *Nagoya J. Med. Sci.* **2009**, *71*, 29.
33. Van Nguyen, H.; Than, P.Q.T.; Nguyen, T.H.; Vu, G.T.; Hoang, C.L.; Tran, T.T.; Truong, N.T.; Nguyen, S.H.; Do, H.P.; Ha, G.H.; et al. Knowledge, Attitude and Practice about Dengue Fever among Patients Experiencing the 2017 Outbreak in Vietnam. *Int. J. Environ. Res. Public Health* **2019**, *16*, 976. [CrossRef]
34. Kai, L.Y.; Yu, C.Y.; Yee, K.P.; Abdullah, S.N.; Hang, T.Q.; Yusop, M.S.; Rahimi, A.; Ismail, F.Z.; Farid, N.D.N.; How, L.S.; et al. Perceptions, attitudes, and responses to dengue early warning among urban community in Kuala Lumpur. *Int. J. Environ. Res. Public Health* **2019**, *19*, 149–159. [CrossRef]
35. Chellaiyan, V.G.; Manoharan, A.; Ramachandran, M. Knowledge and Awareness towards Dengue Infection and Its Prevention: A Cross Sectional Study from Rural Area of Tamil Nadu, India. *Int. J. Community Med. Public Health* **2017**, *4*, 494–499. [CrossRef]
36. Phuyal, P.; Kramer, I.M.; Kuch, U.; Magdeburg, A.; Groneberg, D.A.; Lamichhane Dhimal, M.; Montag, D.; Harapan, H.; Wouters, E.; Jha, A.K.; et al. The Knowledge, Attitude and Practice of Community People on Dengue Fever in Central Nepal: A Cross-Sectional Study. *BMC Infect. Dis.* **2022**, *22*, 454. [CrossRef]
37. Alyousefi, T.A.A.; Abdul-Ghani, R.; Mahdy, M.A.K.; Al-Eryani, S.M.A.; Al-Mekhlafi, A.M.; Raja, Y.A.; Shah, S.A.; Beier, J.C. A Household-Based Survey of Knowledge, Attitudes and Practices towards Dengue Fever among Local Urban Communities in Taiz Governorate, Yemen. *BMC Infect. Dis.* **2016**, *16*, 543. [CrossRef]
38. Ching, S.M.; Ramachandran, V.; Gew, L.T.; Lim, S.M.S.; Sulaiman, W.A.W.; Foo, Y.L.; Zakaria, Z.A.; Samsudin, N.H.; Lau, P.C.M.C.; Veettil, S.K.; et al. Complementary Alternative Medicine Use among Patients with Dengue Fever in the Hospital Setting: A Cross-Sectional Study in Malaysia. *BMC Complement. Altern. Med.* **2016**, *16*, 37. [CrossRef] [PubMed]
39. Khun, S.; Manderson, L. Community and School-Based Health Education for Dengue Control in Rural Cambodia: A Process Evaluation. *PLoS Negl. Trop. Dis.* **2007**, *1*, 143. [CrossRef] [PubMed]
40. Ibrahim, N.K.; Abalkhail, B.; Rady, M.; Al-Bar, H. An educational programme on dengue fever prevention and control for females in Jeddah high schools. *East. Mediterr. Health J.* **2009**, *15*, 1058–1067. [CrossRef] [PubMed]

Tropical Medicine and Infectious Disease

MDPI

Article

Baseline Seroprevalence of Arboviruses in Liberia Using a Multiplex IgG Immunoassay

Albert To [1,*], Varney M. Kamara [1,2], Davidetta M. Tekah [2], Mohammed A. Jalloh [2], Salematu B. Kamara [2], Teri Ann S. Wong [1], Aquena H. Ball [1], Ludwig I. Mayerlen [1], Kyle M. Ishikawa [3], Hyeong Jun Ahn [3], Bode Shobayo [4], Julius Teahton [4], Brien K. Haun [1,5], Wei-Kung Wang [1], John M. Berestecky [1,2,6], Vivek R. Nerurkar [1], Peter S. Humphrey [2] and Axel T. Lehrer [1,*]

1 Department of Tropical Medicine, Medical Microbiology and Pharmacology, John A. Burns School of Medicine, University of Hawai'i at Mānoa, Honolulu, HI 96813, USA
2 Department of Biological Sciences, Medical Science, T.J.R Faulkner College of Science and Technology, University of Liberia, Fendall 1000, Liberia
3 Department of Quantitative Health Sciences, John A. Burns School of Medicine, University of Hawai'i at Mānoa, Honolulu, HI 96813, USA
4 National Public Health Institute of Liberia, Monrovia 1000, Liberia
5 Cell and Molecular Biology Graduate Program, John A. Burns School of Medicine, University of Hawai'i at Mānoa, Honolulu, HI 96813, USA
6 Math & Science Department, Kapiolani Community College, University of Hawai'i at Mānoa, Honolulu, HI 96816, USA
* Correspondence: albertto@hawaii.edu (A.T.); lehrer@hawaii.edu (A.T.L.)

Abstract: Insect-borne viruses may account for a significant proportion of non-malaria and non-bacterial febrile illnesses in Liberia. Although the presence of many arthropod vectors has been documented, the collective burden of arbovirus infections and baseline pre-existing immunity remains enigmatic. Our goal was to determine the seroprevalence of arbovirus exposure across the country using a resource-sparing, multiplex immunoassay to determine IgG responses to immunodominant antigens. 532 human serum samples, from healthy adults, collected from 10 counties across Liberia, were measured for IgG reactivity against antigens of eight common flavi-, alpha-, and orthobunya/nairoviruses suspected to be present in West Africa. Approximately 32.5% of our samples were reactive to alphavirus (CHIKV) E2, ~7% were reactive separately to West Nile (WNV) and Zika virus (ZIKV) NS1, while 4.3 and 3.2% were reactive to Rift Valley Fever virus (RVFV) N and Dengue virus-2 (DENV-2) NS1, respectively. Altogether, 21.6% of our samples were reactive to $\geq$1 flavivirus NS1s. Of the CHIKV E2 reactive samples, 8.5% were also reactive to at least one flavivirus NS1, and six samples were concurrently reactive to antigens of all three arbovirus groups, suggesting a high burden of multiple arbovirus infections for some participants. These insights suggest the presence of these four arbovirus families in Liberia with low and moderate rates of flavi- and alphavirus infections, respectively, in healthy adults. Further confirmational investigation, such as mosquito surveillance or other serological tests, is warranted and should be conducted before initiating additional flavivirus vaccination campaigns. The findings of these studies can help guide healthcare resource mobilization, vector control, and animal husbandry practices.

Keywords: arbovirus; cross-reactivity; IgG; Liberia; microsphere immunoassay; serosurveillance

1. Introduction

The country of Liberia is situated on the lower southwestern tip of West Africa with a population of approximately 5.3 million people living within 15 counties covering

111,370 sq. km. It borders the North Atlantic Ocean to the west, and neighbors Sierra Leone, Guinea, and Côte d'Ivoire [1]. Emerging from more than a decade of civil wars and the recent 2014–15 Ebola virus outbreak, the country is actively engaged in implementing infrastructural improvements to its public health sectors to better manage future biothreats [2]. As part of the pandemic preparedness strategy, active surveillance for human pathogens is being conducted to construct current circulation patterns and natural histories of viral infections in the country. Such comprehensive studies are crucial for guiding government policies, mobilizing healthcare resources, and advising animal husbandry practices in the event of an outbreak.

Given the high number of arbovirus infections in West African nations, mosquito- and tickborne viruses may account for a large proportion of non-malaria and non-bacterial febrile illnesses in Liberia. Such etiologies are severely under-reported as they are frequently undiagnosed, misdiagnosed, or not recognized if asymptomatic [3,4]. The last documented serological study in Liberia, published in 1986, noted a seropositivity rate of 16 and 22% arbovirus-specific antibodies in both epilepsy patients and control participants, respectively [5]. No countrywide survey for common arboviruses has been conducted in Liberia since before the Liberian civil wars. In addition to *Anopheles* sp., many competent *Aedes* and *Culex* sp. vectors are found in Liberia [6]. Considering that the level of urbanization has reached 53% [7] and land use reform has resulted in a deforestation rate of 2% per year prior to 2018 [8], significant landscape changes may contribute to the distribution/adaptation of arbovirus vectors into new habitats, thus expanding the region where the vectors, and the viruses they carry, are found. As mosquito- and tickborne viruses have different lifecycles and reservoir hosts, the ecological niche of these viruses will likely vary across different Liberian counties, from urban and rural communities to coastline regions and neighborhoods bordering other countries.

The purpose of our study is to document the distribution of eight major arboviruses by serology: West Nile virus (WNV), Usutu virus (USUV), Yellow Fever virus (YFV), Dengue virus-2 (DENV-2), Zika virus (ZIKV), Chikungunya virus (CHIKV), Rift Valley Fever virus (RVFV), and Crimean-Congo Hemorrhagic Fever virus (CCHFV). The nonstructural protein 1 (NS1) from the flaviviruses, the envelope 2 protein (E2) from CHIKV, the nucleoprotein (N) from RVFV and glycoprotein c (Gc) from CCHFV were selected as analytes for our multiplex immunoassay (MIA) panel due to their immunodominance leading to high assay sensitivity and virus specificity [9–11]. Serum samples used in this study represent 10 different counties with varying levels of urbanization, spanning the most populous cities to more rural/forest-covered regions of the country. Additionally, seven collection sites share borders with three other West African countries, which provides valuable information on the regional distribution of these arboviruses.

2. Materials and Methods

2.1. Ethical Statement and Sample Collection

Protocols for this study were reviewed and approved by the Institutional Review Boards of the University of Hawai'i at Mānoa, the University of Liberia, as well as the National Research Ethics Review Board of Liberia (NREB). All work was conducted in accordance with institutional and governmental guidelines and regulations. De-identified, archived samples (n = 193) were previously collected from consented, healthy adults (18–80 years of age) in the four counties most heavily affected by the 2014/2015 Ebola Virus Disease outbreak: Montserrado, Margibi, Grand Bassa, and Bong. Additional archived human blood samples (n = 200), from a Lassa Fever study, originating in Bong, Lofa, Nimba, and Grand Bassa county, as well as prospective samples (n = 199) from Grand Cape Mount, Gbarpolu, Grand Gedeh, and River Gee county, were also tested. Approximately 5–10 mL of blood was drawn by venipuncture into BD vacutainer tiger top tubes (BD, Accra, Ghana) from each participant. Sera were separated onsite by centrifugation at 1000–2000× g for 10 min and aliquoted into cryovial tubes prior to immediate freezing in a mobile −80 °C freezer. Samples were transported at temperatures below −20 °C to the University of Liberia Fendall Mobile Laboratory for storage at −80 °C until analysis.

2.2. Antigen

Stably transformed cell lines expressing the flavivirus (USUV [strain SAAR-1774], DENV-2 [strain TSV01], and ZIKV [strain H/FP/2013]) NS1 and alphavirus (CHIKV [strain Senegal 37997] E2 were generated, generally as previously described [12,13]. Briefly, codon-optimized synthetic genes (IDT, Coralville, IA; and Twist Biosciences, San Francisco, CA, USA) were inserted downstream of an inducible metallothionein (MT) promoter in plasmid vectors pMT-BiP (Invitrogen, Waltham, WA, USA) or pUHM (proprietary). Drosophila S2 cells were transfected with the appropriate selection marker using Lipofectamine-based transfection reagents (Invitrogen, Carlsbad, CA, USA) and cultured in the presence of hygromycin (InvivoGen, San Diego, CA, USA) until stable cell growth was observed. Cell lines were induced with 200 μM copper sulfate, and antigen expression was determined using SDS-PAGE and immunoblot using a 6x-his-tag secondary antibody (Thermofisher Scientific, Waltham, WA, USA).

Recombinant antigens were purified from clarified cell culture supernatants using a HisTrap FF column (Cytiva, Marlborough, MA, USA). Optimized purification protocols, using a single or double imidazole elution step, were developed for each antigen to achieve maximum purity. Select fractions containing the antigen were pooled, buffer-exchanged into PBS, and stored at −80 °C until use. Purity for all internally produced antigens was ≥90% as estimated by SDS-PAGE.

Drosophila S2-expressed WNV NS1 and CCHFV Gc were gifted by Hawai'i Biotech Inc. (Honolulu, HI, USA), and YFV NS1 (cat no. YFV-NS1-100) and RVFV N (cat no. REC31640-100) were purchased from the Native Antigen Company (Oxford, UK). The reactivity of each antigen was confirmed using a panel of arbovirus IgG reference sera (provided by the Vector Borne Disease Branch of the US Centers for Disease Control and Prevention, and the United States Department of Agriculture) by Western blot.

2.3. Arbovirus Microsphere Panel

Antigens were coupled to spectrally distinct MagPlex-C Microspheres (Luminex Corporation, Austin, TX, USA) using a modified, two-step carbodiimide reaction based on the manufacturer's protocol. A total of 25 μg of each antigen was covalently coupled to the surface of 5×10^6 microspheres. The antigen-conjugated microspheres were stored in 800 μL of PBS-TBN buffer (PBS with 0.1% bovine serum albumin Fraction V, 0.02% Tween-20, and 0.01% sodium azide (Sigma-Aldrich, St. Louis, MO, USA) at 2–8 °C until use.

2.4. Microsphere Immunoassay

IgG seroreactivity of human serum samples to each of the eight arbovirus antigens and BSA as the negative antigen control was measured using a multiplex microsphere-based immunoassay (MIA) as described previously [13]. The MagPix instrument was calibrated with reference beads prior to each use. Serum samples were initially diluted to 1:100 with PBS+ 1% BSA and 0.02% Tween 20 (PBS-BT) and added to the arbovirus microsphere panel (1:200 suspended in PBS-BT) 1:1 in black-sided 96-well plates in duplicates. The antibody-bead complex was allowed to form for 3 h at ambient temperature (32–35 °C) with agitation. After two PBS-BT wash steps, 50 μL of 1 μg/mL red phycoerythrin (R-PE)-conjugated goat anti-human IgG antibodies (Jackson ImmunoResearch, Inc., West Grove, PA, USA) were added to each well and incubated at ambient temperature with agitation for 1 h. Finally, after another series of wash steps and resuspension in MAGPIX® drive fluid, the median fluorescence intensity (MFI) was measured using a MAGPIX® Instrument (Luminex Corporation, Austin, TX, USA). Samples with coefficient of variation percent (CV%) values of >15% or with low bead counts (below 50 beads per region) were retested.

2.5. Statistical Analysis

Samples with high background, i.e., a MFI of 1500 or greater for BSA and all other analytes, were removed from further analysis. MFI cutoff for high seroreactivity was determined using a Gaussian mixture model to identify clustering of low, medium, and high MFIs [14]. Values were log-transformed, and the maximum likelihood estimation for normal clusters of a specified number of components was determined using the Expectation-Maximization (EM) algorithm within the (mixR) package on R software (v 4.3.1) [15]. The number of components for each distribution was increased until a clear high MFI cluster was distinguishable. The vertical intercept between the left tail of the high MFI and the right tail of the adjacent normal curves was set as the cutoff for highly seroreactive samples (Figure S1A). The assay background was determined using the mean MFI of BSA + 3 standard deviations. Individual antigen analyte cutoffs of low-medium seroreactivity were determined using the mean MFI of samples showing no specific reactivity to any analyte + 3 standard deviations. Although not available for every analyte, the cutoff demarcating highly seroreactive samples was verified using positive reference sera.

To resolve the signal interference caused by cross-reactivity between the USUV, WNV, YFV, DENV-2, and ZIKV NS1s, ratios for each analyte were generated by dividing each of the flavivirus NS1 MFIs by the NS1 MFIs of interest for each participant sample [9]. This yielded a single relative MFI (rMFI) ratio of 1.0, where the numerator and denominator values are the same analyte, and four other ratios of either <1.0 or >1.0 for the other flavivirus NS1 analytes (Figure S1B). Samples with monotypic reactivity for a single flavivirus NS1 had a ratio of 1.0 for the analyte corresponding to the probable etiology of the primary infection and had relative ratios of <0.5 for the other four flavivirus NS1 analytes. Samples with reactivity to two or more flavivirus NS1s, defined as having two rMFI ratios $\geq$ 1.0, were categorized as having had multiple flavivirus infections. To determine the distribution of flavivirus infections by county (Table 1), only the strongest flavivirus NS1 response was considered. In the case of samples having multiple NS1 reactivities above the established cutoff, the NS1 analyte with the highest MFI was selected, while the other NS1 MFI values were removed from the tally. Only a single NS1 analyte contributed to the final count. Samples with multiple flavivirus NS1 rMFI ratios >1 were enumerated and counted separately (Table 2).

Graphical representation was plotted using Prism, GraphPad Software (v10.0.1), (San Diego, CA, USA).

3. Results

Archived samples from 393 healthy adult participants from Montserrado, Margibi, Grand Bassa, Bong, Nimba, and Lofa counties were collected in 2021 to survey the seroprevalence of Ebola and Lassa virus after the 2014 Ebola Virus Disease and annual Lassa Fever outbreaks. To gain greater resolution and to provide a contrast to the urban counties with large population centers (Figure 1A), 199 samples were prospectively collected from participants inhabiting Grand Cape Mount, Gbarpolu, Grand Gedeh, and River Gee counties. These four counties are comprised primarily of rural communities, with lower population densities, and border the countries of Sierra Leone, Guinea, and Côte d'Ivoire (Figure 1A,B).

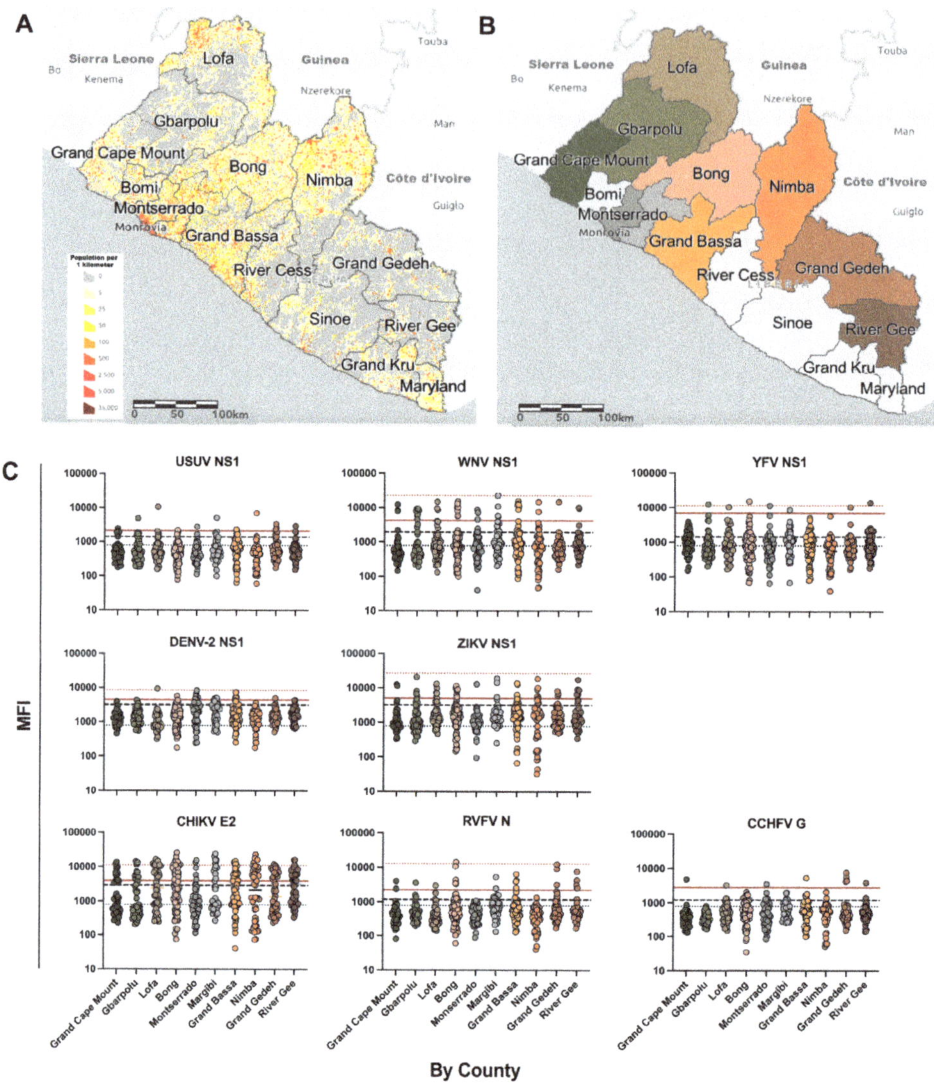

Figure 1. Distribution of arbovirus seroreactivity in 10 counties across Liberia. (**A**) Population distribution of Liberia per square kilometer. The image was generated with ArcGIS Online, using the 2016 Liberian Population Density layer, generated by the USAID Liberia, available on the online service. (**B**) Selected counties where participant serum samples originated. Each selected county is displayed in a different color. (**C**) Curated distribution of arbovirus antigen reactivities by county. The black dotted line indicates the background signal of BSA + 3 STDEV. The black dashed line indicates the analyte-specific assay cutoff determined by using the mean MFI of samples showing no specific reactivity to any analyte + 3 STDEV. The red solid line indicates the Gaussian mixture model cutoff for highly seroreactive samples. Where available, the red dotted line indicates the MFI value of a PCR-confirmed, arbovirus-positive reference sera.

Table 1. Individual Count, Percentage by County and Countrywide Total of Highly Seroreactive Samples to Each Arbovirus Antigen.

County	n	USUV NS1	WNV NS1	YFV NS1	DENV-2 NS1	ZIKV NS1	RVFV N	CHIKV E2	CCHFV Gc
Grand Cape Mount	49	1 (2.0%)	3 (6.1%)	-	-	2 (4.1%)	2 (4.1%)	13 (26.5%)	1 (2.0%)
Gbarpolu	50	1 (2.0%)	9 (18.0%)	1 (2.0%)	-	4 (8.0%)	1 (2.0%)	12 (24.0%)	-
Lofa	50	1 (2.0%)	3 (6.0%)	1 (2.0%)	1 (2.0%)	5 (10.0%)	1 (2.0%)	22 (44.0%)	1 (2.0%)
Bong	79	1 (1.3%)	8 (10.1%)	1 (1.3%)	1 (2.0%)	5 (6.3%)	5 (6.3%)	29 (36.7%)	-
Montserrado	51	1 (2.0%)	3 (5.9%)	1 (2.0%)	7 (13.7%)	1 (2.0%)	-	5 (9.0%)	1 (2.0%)
Margibi	40	1 (2.5%)	4 (10.0%)	1 (2.5%)	2 (5.0%)	3 (7.5%)	2 (5.0%)	11 (27.5%)	-
Grand Bassa	66	1 (1.5%)	6 (9.1%)	-	4 (6.1%)	3 (4.5%)	4 (6.1%)	20 (30.3%)	1 (1.5%)
Nimba	48	1 (2.1%)	2 (4.2%)	-	-	6 (12.5%)	-	21 (43.8%)	-
Grand Gedeh	49	3 (6.1%)	1 (2.0%)	1 (2.0%)	1 (2.0%)	4 (8.2%)	3 (6.1%)	17 (34.7.0%)	4 (8.2%)
River Gee	50	1 (2.0%)	2 (4.0%)	1 (2.0%)	1 (2.0%)	5 (10.0%)	5 (10.0%)	23 (46.0%)	1 (2.0%)
Countrywide Total	532	12	41	7	17	38	23	173	9
Percentage	-	2.3%	7.7%	1.3%	3.2%	7.1%	4.3%	32.5%	1.7%

- indicates no seroreactivity detected.

Table 2. Probable count, percentage by county, and countrywide total of single and multiple arbovirus infections.

County	n	Single Flavivirus Infection	Multiple (≥2) Flavivirus Infections	Total Flavivirus Infection	Single Flavivirus w/CHIKV Infection	Multiple Flavivirus w/CHIKV Infection	CHIKV with RVFV Infection	CHIKV with CCHFV Infection
Grand Cape Mount	49	6 (12.2%)	-	6 (12.2%)	2 (4.1%)	-	-	-
Gbarpolu	50	13 (26.0%)	2 (4.0%)	15 (30.0%)	6 (12.0%)	-	1 (2.0%)	-
Lofa	50	9 (18.0%)	2 (4.0%)	11 (22.0%)	4 (8.0%)	-	1^s (2.0%)	-
Bong	79	11 (13.9%)	5 (6.3%)	16 (20.3%)	8 (10.1%)	4 (5.1%)	3 (1^s) (3.8%)	-
Montserrado	51	12 (23.5%)	1 (2.0%)	13 (25.5%)	1 (2.0%)	1 (2.0%)	-	1^m (2.0%)
Margibi	40	7 (17.5%)	4 (10.0%)	11 (27.5%)	-	2 (5.0%)	1 (2.5%)	-
Grand Bassa	66	11 (16.7%)	3 (4.5%)	14 (21.2%)	4 (6.1%)	2 (3.0%)	-	1^m (1.5%)
Nimba	48	9 (18.8%)	-	9 (18.8%)	4 (8.3%)	-	-	-
Grand Gedeh	49	7 (14.3%)	3 (6.1%)	10 (20.4%)	2 (4.1%)	2 (4.1%)	-	3 (6.1%)
River Gee	50	10 (20.0%)	-	10 (20.0%)	3 (6.0%)	-	2 (1^s) (4.0%)	1^s (2.0%)
Countrywide Total	532	95	20	115	34	11	8	6
Percentage	-	17.9%	3.8%	21.6%	6.4%	2.1%	1.5%	1.1%

- indicates no seroreactivity detected. n^s indicates the number of people with a single flavivirus infection and n^m indicates the number of people with multiple flavivirus infections with CHIKV and either RVFV or CCHFV infections.

Of the 592 serum samples tested, 60 samples were removed from the analysis due to excessively high background signals and non-specific binding to all analytes, including BSA, which is used as a negative analyte control and is present in all assay buffers. Samples removed from the analysis showed either signs of hemolysis or had high lipid content; however, a few samples were aberrantly reactive without any visible signs of compromised sample integrity. A total of 532 samples yielded consistent MFI values with a low background signal. Gaussian mixture modeling of log-transformed MFI values was used to identify low, medium, and high MFI clusters that were used to establish cutoffs distinguishing highly seroreactive samples apart from adjacent lower MFI clusters (Figure S1A). Samples with MFIs greater than the cutoff value were considered highly seroreactive and likely to have antigen-specific antibodies for the detected analyte.

Cross-reactivity between the flavivirus NS1s (homology ranging from 45 to 76%), which yields MFIs above the set cutoffs for multiple flavivirus analytes, could result in duplicate counting. This was controlled for by using rMFI ratios, where the MFI of each flavivirus NS1 analyte is divided by the MFI of the NS1 of interest (Figure S1B). Reactivity to a single NS1 analyte indicates that a participant has had only a primary flavivirus infection, whereas reactivity to two or more NS1 analytes suggests multiple flavivirus infections. Table 1 displays the total count of sample reactivities to all arbovirus analytes countrywide and sorted by county. Here, only the tally of single flavivirus was counted. In the event a serum sample is reactive to two or more flavivirus NS1s, the analyte with the highest ratio was selected for the final count, and its corresponding MFI readouts for the other flavivirus NS1s were removed from the tally.

Overall, a third of our serum samples (32.5%) were reactive to the CHIKV E2, suggesting a moderate seroprevalence for alphaviruses in the Liberian population. This was followed by reactivities to WNV NS1 at 7.7% and ZIKV NS1 at 7.1%. Lower seroprevalence was observed for RVFV N at 4.3% and DENV-2 NS1 at 3.2%. While at much lower rates, IgG against USUV NS1, YFV NS1, and CCHFV Gc were also detected. The presence of these antigen-specific antibodies suggests that at least eight arboviruses may have or are currently circulating in Liberia.

Table 2 displays the count of samples with single flavivirus and multiple arbovirus reactivity. Approximately 17.9% of our samples were reactive to only a single flavivirus analyte, while 3.8% were reactive to two or more flavivirus NS1s. Co-reactivities for both DENV-2 and ZIKV NS1s were the most common. Altogether, over a fifth of our samples (21.6%) were reactive to at least one flavivirus NS1. Of the samples reactive to CHIKV E2, 6.4% and 2.1% were also reactive to either a single or multiple flavivirus NS1(s), respectively, for a total of 8.5% co-exposure. Similarly, approximately 1–2% of CHIKV E2 reactive samples were also reactive to either RVFV N or CCHFV Gc, and six samples were reactive to at least one analyte from three virus families with no pattern based on location.

4. Discussion

This report provides the first published update on the epidemiological situation of arbovirus infections in Liberia since 1986 [5]. Our pilot study uses a multiplex immunoassay based on serum reactivity to immunodominant, recombinant antigen from eight highly relevant arboviruses, and a statistical modeling approach using MFI signal clustering, to determine if the spatial differences in arbovirus antigen reactivity can be seen in 532 archived and prospective serum samples collected from 10 counties.

Overall, arbovirus infections appear to be widespread throughout the country. Approximately 60% of our samples were reactive to at least one arbovirus analyte. Notably, there is a moderate to low degree of alphavirus and flavivirus seroprevalence. The most prevalent infection appears to be from an alphavirus (CHIKV), followed by WNV, ZIKV, RVFV and finally DENV-2; altogether suggesting endemic circulation of these arboviruses in Liberia. There is also a low rate of dual reactivity to antigens from both alphaviruses and flaviviruses in some samples; with six samples reactive to antigens of three arbovirus families, indicating a potentially heavy burden of mosquito-borne diseases for a few individuals. After accounting for possible cross-reactivity, evidence of YFV, USUV, and CCHFV infections was found, with approximately one sample per county, with some exceptions, seroreactive to these antigens; however, it is not clear whether this indicates active endemic transmission rather than cross-border transmission from neighboring countries [16–18]. The primary vectors for all these arboviruses (*Aedes aegypti*, *Culex pipiens*, *Hyalomma* spp., respectively) are present in Liberia [6,19].

The arboviral landscape of Liberia reported here aligns with large-scale, mosquito-borne disease outbreaks and serological evidence of flavi-, alpha-, and orthobunya-/nairoviruses documented in this region [20–31]. Antibodies to CHIKV have been reported in individuals from Liberia and Sierra Leone since 1977 [32], and was cited as a cause of acute febrile illnesses in Sierra Leone [30] and Guinea [33]. Our report of 32.5% seroprevalence for CHIKV is consistent with the 31.2% reported in Mali [34], and the 38.5–54% reported in Senegal [35,36]. CHIKV E2 reactivity may also be attributed to, or at least in part, by O'nyong'nyong virus (ONNV), a closely related but divergent alphavirus, transmitted by *Anopheles* mosquitoes [37]. The E2 antigen of CHIKV and ONNV shares 87% homology. Neutralization tests performed with ONNV on CHIKV IgM+ samples in Sierra Leone suggest that ONNV may be predominant in West Africa [30], and a 2003 outbreak in neighboring Côte d'Ivoire makes this notion highly plausible that ONNV cross-reactivity may contribute to the high rate of CHIKV E2 reactivity in our assay [38]. While we attempted to include ONNV E2 in our analysis, the purity of our antigen was ~25%, which resulted in a high background signal in our assay. Together with the high homology, we could not establish a clear antigen cutoff and thus excluded the ONNV data set from our final analysis.

By contrast, the IgG seroprevalence to WNV (7.7%) and ZIKV (7.1%) NS1s in our samples are lower than the rates reported in other countries; however, many of the seroprevalence rates reported in the literature are derived from febrile or clinic-based patient samples and cannot be directly compared. The prevalence rates of WNV antibodies in febrile patients in Mali were reported to be 39% [39], and upwards of 40% in Sierra Leone [40]. In healthy children and adults in Ghana, the rate of WNV-specific IgG was ~30% overall. By comparison, ZIKV seroprevalence in Mali was 12% [41] and 25.8% [34] for afebrile and febrile participants, respectively, while the average IgM seroprevalence of febrile patients in Guinea was about 14.7% [42].

While RVFV has been detected in animals in Senegal, Guinea, and Côte d'Ivoire [43–46], the prevalence of infection in humans appears to vary depending on the region sampled [47] and on the occupation of the individual, with higher infection rates found in those working with livestock [48]. The overall seroprevalence of RVFV in Africa was reported as 7.9% [49] and is comparable to our rate of 4.3%.

Molecular evidence of all four DENV serotypes has been recorded in Senegal, Burkina Faso, Ghana, Sierra Leone, and Côte d'Ivoire, where the viruses are endemic [20,31,50–55]. Similarly, much of the seroprevalence of DENV reported in the literature is derived from febrile patients; however, the distribution of these infections is likely heterogeneous depending on the region sampled [56]. Between 69.2 and 78.6% of febrile hospital patients in Ghana and Sierra Leone were determined to have been infected with DENV [57,58]. One study in Mali, via random household sampling, reported a seroprevalence rate of 77.2% based on virus neutralization tests [34]. Comparatively, the DENV-2 NS1 seroprevalence rate of 3.2% in our study is much lower. The higher rates for flavivirus NS1 reactivity in the literature could be partially attributed to the difficulty in distinguishing flavivirus cross-reactivity, especially in the case of multiple flavivirus infections, using commercial ELISA kits. Furthermore, our DENV NS1 analyte, derived from DENV-2, may not capture the full extent of all DENV serotype infections, especially from low-titer convalescent samples.

It is evident, though, that highly DENV-2 NS1 reactive samples appeared to largely cluster in the central coastal counties of Liberia with the majority coming from Montserrado and Grand Bassa counties, which have urban or semi-urban settings along the Atlantic Ocean. The lower coastal elevation, slightly warmer climate, and contribution of salinity-adapted *Aedes aegypti* may explain the urban distribution of DENV-2 observed in this study [59,60]. This mosquito species is the primary vector for DENV and is found commonly in anthropophilic settings [6]. It is also noted that no RVFV N reactive samples were detected from Montserrado County, which supports the observation that RVFV is primarily a rural disease [61]. While both *Aedes* and *Culex* spp. are susceptible to RVFV infection, transmission by *Aedes aegypti* appears to be host-dependent [61,62] and unlikely in an urban setting, as ruminant hosts are less likely to be present [61]. Similarly, CHIKV reactive samples were more prevalent outside of Montserrado County and may be attributed to the greater presence of *Aedes albopictus,* which is typically found in rural settings [63], and is a more competent vector for CHIKV than *Aedes aegypti* [64]. The dichotomy of DENV-2 and CHIKV seroprevalence may be explained by the preferred habitats of these two *Aedes* spp. [65]. Although less prominent, a similar trend was observed with ZIKV infections, as only a single reactive sample originated in Montserrado County. The contribution of CHIKV and ZIKV transmission from the sylvatic cycle by *Aedes albopictus* and *Aedes africanus* is a possible factor for their predominance in rural settings [25,66]. In terms of total flavivirus infections, there appears to be an even spread across the country, whereas individuals with both flavivirus and alphavirus (CHIKV) infection appear more frequently outside the urbanized Montserrado and Margibi counties. Lastly, there is a trend of more WNV infections occurring west of Nimba County. Although *Aedes* spp. are competent vectors for WNV transmission, *Culex* spp., especially *Culex quinquefasciatus*, predominate as the primary source of transmission in Africa [67]. This seroprevalence pattern suggests that the distribution of arboviruses may be determined by the type of mosquito hosts that inhabit certain ecological niches created by terrain, climate, and level of urbanization.

Precautions were taken to ensure valid measurements and accurate classification within our data set, however, there are some limitations to be considered. (1) A portion of samples, especially those archived, were deidentified or lost, and thus, sociodemographic data could not be analyzed to establish potential risk factors. (2) Systematic household sampling was not possible in every circumstance; thus, a portion of sera were collected on a voluntary basis at a single community center in the county. This sampling bias could subtly influence our results, as some samples were collected only from those who could travel to the collection site. However, our non-healthcare-based sample pool of healthy adults may capture asymptomatic and underreported cases that would otherwise be missed. (3) Although most of our samples yielded clear readouts with low background interference, we had to exclude some samples during our quality control screening due to poor sample integrity. This reduced our sample size by 10%. Timely sample processing is critical for settings where access to laboratory equipment is not feasible within a few hours after collection. It is recommended that blood samples be processed as soon as possible and immediately transported/stored between −20 and to −80 °C. (4) Our assay relied on IgG reactivity to immunodominant antigens. While this enables better specificity compared to traditional ELISA methods and allows for evaluation of antibody binding in the context of other similar antigens, NS1 cross-reactivity still limits the resolution required to distinguish the etiology of multiple flavivirus infections. Virus neutralization tests will be required to corroborate our results; however, this is exceedingly difficult to accomplish in-country due to the lack of appropriately equipped biocontainment facilities, assay reagents, and skilled personnel. The utility of this microsphere immunoassay stems from its high-throughput capacity to quickly and widely survey for the presence of antibodies in humans or animals [68] against certain pathogens as routine disease surveillance or in response to an outbreak situation. As IgG binding-based assays are not as definitive as neutralization tests, the addition of *Aedes* and *Culex* spp. to ongoing mosquito surveillance can help corroborate the presence of these specific arboviruses in the country. (5) Lastly, our YFV NS1 analyte is unable to discriminate wt-YFV infection from responses generated with vaccination-attenuated YFV-17D. While the countrywide YF vaccination coverage had dropped below 60% between 2014 and 2015, current coverage is estimated to be ~78–92% in 2022. Our results can only be interpreted as baseline YFV immunity rather than the prevalence of YFV infections.

5. Conclusions

Our analysis provides a critical update of baseline arbovirus immunity in Liberia. We show low and moderate rates of flavi- and alphavirus infections, respectively, in healthy adults, with more DENV-2 seroprevalence in urban counties and ZIKV and CHIKV seroprevalence in rural counties. The seroreactivity rates for RVFV and CCHFV are also low relative to other African countries. This alludes to the role of various mosquito vectors in arbovirus distribution, thus careful speciation of *Aedes*, *Culex*, and *Anopheles* (for ONNV) mosquitos may provide further insight into virus transmission patterns. Arbovirus-specific confirmational tests and/or mosquito surveillance should be conducted before the initiation of mass vaccination campaigns in the country. The findings of these studies can further help guide healthcare resource mobilization, vector control, and animal husbandry practices.

Supplementary Materials: The following supporting information can be downloaded at: https://www.mdpi.com/article/10.3390/tropicalmed10040092/s1, Figure S1: Distribution of Arboviruses in 10 Counties across Liberia.

Author Contributions: Conceptualization, A.T., V.M.K., J.M.B., V.R.N., P.S.H. and A.T.L.; methodology, A.T., V.M.K., D.M.T., M.A.J., S.B.K., T.A.S.W., A.H.B., L.I.M. and B.K.H.; formal analysis, A.T., V.M.K., K.M.I., H.J.A., W.-K.W. and A.T.L.; investigation, A.T., V.M.K., D.M.T., M.A.J., S.B.K., P.S.H. and A.T.L.; resources, A.T., V.M.K., D.M.T., M.A.J., S.B.K., B.S., J.T., J.M.B., V.R.N., P.S.H. and A.T.L.; data curation, A.T., K.M.I. and H.J.A.; writing—original draft preparation, A.T.; writing—review and editing, all authors; visualization, A.T. and K.M.I.; supervision, A.T., V.M.K., J.M.B., V.R.N., P.S.H. and A.T.L.; project administration, A.T., V.M.K., J.M.B., V.R.N., P.S.H. and A.T.L.; funding acquisition, A.T., V.R.N., P.S.H. and A.T.L. All authors have read and agreed to the published version of the manuscript.

Funding: Funding for this project was provided by the Robert E. Shope International Fellowship from the American Society of Tropical Medicine and Hygiene. Funding was also provided, in part, by a Cooperative Agreement (U01-GH-002256) between the Centers for Disease Control and Prevention and the University of Hawaii, the Ola HAWAII Program, PIKO and support facilities (U54MD007601 and U54GM138062) and the Minority Health Research Training Program (T37MD008636) from the National Institute on Minority Health and Health Disparities, a research grant from the National Institute of Allergy and Infectious Diseases (R01AI132323), and the Northern Pacific Global Health Fellowship Program (D43TW009345) from the Fogarty International Center, National Institutes of Health (NIH).

Institutional Review Board Statement: Serum samples for the described studies in Liberia were collected under a protocol approved by the National Research Ethics Board (NREB) protocol number NREB-018-20 and by the University of Liberia Institutional Review Board protocol number UL-IRB/JCT-CH/039/'22 (approved 12 December 2022).

Informed Consent Statement: Informed consent was obtained from all subjects involved in the study.

Data Availability Statement: Date will be provided upon reasonable request by the corresponding authors, Albert To (albertto@hawaii.edu), and Axel T. Lehrer (lehrer@hawaii.edu).

Acknowledgments: We would like to thank David Clements from Hawai'i Biotech Inc. for providing the WNV NS1 and CCHFV Gc antigens used in our arbovirus antigen panel. We would also like to thank Ann M. Powers and Eric C. Mossel from the Vector Borne Disease Branch of the US CDC and William Wilson from the USDA for their scientific support and for providing reference sera or services used to validate several antigens and beads used in this study. Lastly, we would like to acknowledge Sackie Moses, our driver from the University of Liberia, for his vital role during the sample collection, along with the staff of the Liberia Institute of Biomedical Research and our extended family in Liberia for their support. Images from Figure 1A,B. were generated with ArcGIS Online using layers made available on the online service by USAID Liberia.

Conflicts of Interest: The authors have no conflicts of interest to declare. All co-authors have seen and agree with the contents of the manuscript, and there is no financial interest to report. The opinions expressed in this manuscript are the author's own and do not reflect the views of the American Society for Tropical Medicine and Hygiene or the National Institutes of Health.

References

1. Liberia Institute of Statistics and Geo-Information Services. *Liberia Demographic and Health Survey 2019–2020*; Liberia Institute of Statistics and Geo-Information Services (LISGIS): Monrovia, Liberia, 2020.
2. Ndede, P.O.; Senkungu, J.K.; Shakpeh, J.K.; Jones, T.E.; Sky, R.; McDonnell, S. Health Services and Infrastructure Recovery of a Major Public Hospital in Liberia During the 2014–2016 Ebola Epidemic. *Disaster Med. Public Health Prep.* **2019**, *13*, 767–773. [CrossRef] [PubMed]
3. Sow, A.; Loucoubar, C.; Diallo, D.; Faye, O.; Ndiaye, Y.; Senghor, C.S.; Dia, A.T.; Faye, O.; Weaver, S.C.; Diallo, M.; et al. Concurrent malaria and arbovirus infections in Kedougou, southeastern Senegal. *Malar. J.* **2016**, *15*, 47. [CrossRef]
4. Baba, M.; Logue, C.H.; Oderinde, B.; Abdulmaleek, H.; Williams, J.; Lewis, J.; Laws, T.R.; Hewson, R.; Marcello, A.; D'Agaro, P. Evidence of arbovirus co-infection in suspected febrile malaria and typhoid patients in Nigeria. *J. Infect. Dev. Ctries.* **2013**, *7*, 51–59. [CrossRef]
5. Van der Waals, F.W.; Asher, D.M.; Goudsmit, J.; Pomeroy, K.L.; Karabatsos, N.; Gajdusek, D.C. Post-encephalitic epilepsy and arbovirus infections in an isolated rainforest area of central Liberia. *Trop. Geogr. Med.* **1986**, *38*, 203–208. [PubMed]
6. Fox, R.M. Man-biting mosquitoes in coastal Liberia. *Am. J. Trop. Med. Hyg.* **1958**, *7*, 215–220. [CrossRef] [PubMed]
7. Liberia-Country Summary, The World Factbook. Available online: https://www.cia.gov/the-world-factbook/countries/liberia/ (accessed on 2 January 2024).
8. Christensen, D.; Hartman, A.C.; Samii, C. Citizen monitoring promotes informed and inclusive forest governance in Liberia. *Proc. Natl. Acad. Sci. USA* **2021**, *118*, e2015169118. [CrossRef]
9. Tyson, J.; Tsai, W.Y.; Tsai, J.J.; Massgard, L.; Stramer, S.L.; Lehrer, A.T.; Nerurkar, V.R.; Wang, W.K. A high-throughput and multiplex microsphere immunoassay based on non-structural protein 1 can discriminate three flavivirus infections. *PLoS Negl. Trop. Dis.* **2019**, *13*, e0007649. [CrossRef]
10. Surtees, R.; Stern, D.; Ahrens, K.; Kromarek, N.; Lander, A.; Kreher, P.; Weiss, S.; Hewson, R.; Punch, E.K.; Barr, J.N.; et al. Development of a multiplex microsphere immunoassay for the detection of antibodies against highly pathogenic viruses in human and animal serum samples. *PLoS Negl. Trop. Dis.* **2020**, *14*, e0008699. [CrossRef]
11. Belij-Rammerstorfer, S.; Limon, G.; Maze, E.A.; Hannant, K.; Hughes, E.; Tchakarova, S.R.; Alexandrov, T.; Mmbaga, B.T.; Willett, B.; Booth, G.; et al. Development of anti-Crimean-Congo hemorrhagic fever virus Gc and NP-specific ELISA for detection of antibodies in domestic animal sera. *Front. Vet. Sci.* **2022**, *9*, 913046. [CrossRef]
12. To, A.; Medina, L.O.; Mfuh, K.O.; Lieberman, M.M.; Wong, T.A.S.; Namekar, M.; Nakano, E.; Lai, C.Y.; Kumar, M.; Nerurkar, V.R.; et al. Recombinant Zika Virus Subunits Are Immunogenic and Efficacious in Mice. *mSphere* **2018**, *3*, e00576-17. [CrossRef]
13. Haun, B.K.; To, A.; Williams, C.A.; Ball, A.; Fong, K.; Wong, T.A.S.; Shobayo, B.; Teahton, J.; Ching, L.; Kamara, V.; et al. A Serological Multiplexed Immunoassay (MIA) Detects Antibody Reactivity to SARS-CoV-2 and Other Viral Pathogens in Liberia and Is Configurable as a Multiplexed Inhibition Test (MINT). *Immuno* **2024**, *4*, 108–124. [CrossRef] [PubMed]
14. Gay, N.J. Analysis of serological surveys using mixture models: Application to a survey of parvovirus B19. *Stat. Med.* **1996**, *15*, 1567–1573. [CrossRef] [PubMed]
15. Yu, Y. mixR: Finite Mixture Modeling for Raw and Binned Data, R Package Version 0.2.0. 2022. Available online: https://www.theoj.org/joss-papers/joss.04031/10.21105.joss.04031.pdf (accessed on 3 July 2023).
16. Nikolay, B.; Diallo, M.; Boye, C.S.; Sall, A.A. Usutu virus in Africa. *Vector Borne Zoonotic Dis.* **2011**, *11*, 1417–1423. [CrossRef]

17. Pisano, M.R.; Nicoli, J.; Tolou, H. Homogeneity of yellow fever virus strains isolated during an epidemic and a post-epidemic period in West Africa. *Virus Genes* **1997**, *14*, 225–234. [CrossRef]
18. Adjogoua, E.V.; Coulibaly-Guindo, N.; Diaha-Kouame, C.A.; Diane, M.K.; Kouassi, R.; Coulibaly, J.T.; Dosso, M. Geographical Distribution of Ticks Ixodidae in Cote d'Ivoire: Potential Reservoir of the Crimean-Congo Hemorrhagic Fever Virus. *Vector Borne Zoonotic Dis.* **2021**, *21*, 628–634. [CrossRef]
19. Mediannikov, O.; Diatta, G.; Zolia, Y.; Balde, M.C.; Kohar, H.; Trape, J.F.; Raoult, D. Tick-borne rickettsiae in Guinea and Liberia. *Ticks Tick. Borne Dis.* **2012**, *3*, 43–48. [CrossRef] [PubMed]
20. Dieng, I.; Ndiaye, M.; Ndione, M.H.D.; Sankhe, S.; Diagne, M.M.; Sagne, S.N.; Gaye, A.; Balde, D.; Barry, A.; Fall, G.; et al. Molecular characterization of circulating Dengue virus 2 during an outbreak in Northern Senegal's Saint-Louis region in 2018. *J. Med. Virol.* **2023**, *95*, e28347. [CrossRef]
21. Yonga, M.G.; Yandai, F.H.; Sadeuh-Mba, S.; Abdallah, A.H.; Ouapi, D.; Gamougam, K.; Abanda, N.N.; Endengue-Zanga, M.C.; Demanou, M.; Njouom, R. Molecular characterization of chikungunya virus from the first cluster of patients during the 2020 outbreak in Chad. *Arch. Virol.* **2022**, *167*, 1301–1305. [CrossRef]
22. Faye, O.; de Lourdes Monteiro, M.; Vrancken, B.; Prot, M.; Lequime, S.; Diarra, M.; Ndiaye, O.; Valdez, T.; Tavarez, S.; Ramos, J.; et al. Genomic Epidemiology of 2015–2016 Zika Virus Outbreak in Cape Verde. *Emerg. Infect. Dis.* **2020**, *26*, 1084–1090. [CrossRef]
23. Leaders de l'Actualité Africaine. Burkina Faso: 688 Décès Liés à la Dengue Depuis le Début de l'Année. Available online: https://www.faapa.info/blog/burkina-faso-688-deces-lies-a-la-dengue-depuis-le-debut-de-lannee/ (accessed on 2 January 2023).
24. Nigeria Centre for Disease Control and Prevention. NCDC on Alert Following the Confirmation of the Dengue Fever Outbreak in Sokoto State. Available online: https://ncdc.gov.ng/news/506/ncdc-on-alert-following-the-confirmation-of-the-dengue-fever-outbreak-in-sokoto-state (accessed on 2 January 2024).
25. Padane, A.; Tegally, H.; Ramphal, Y.; Seyni, N.; Sarr, M.; Diop, M.M.; Diedhiou, C.K.; Mboup, A.; Diouf, N.D.; Souare, A.; et al. An emerging clade of Chikungunya West African genotype discovered in real-time during 2023 outbreak in Senegal. *medRxiv* **2023**. [CrossRef]
26. Hoze, N.; Diarra, I.; Sangare, A.K.; Pastorino, B.; Pezzi, L.; Kouriba, B.; Sagara, I.; Dabo, A.; Djimde, A.; Thera, M.A.; et al. Model-based assessment of Chikungunya and O'nyong-nyong virus circulation in Mali in a serological cross-reactivity context. *Nat. Commun.* **2021**, *12*, 6735. [CrossRef] [PubMed]
27. Lim, J.K.; Ridde, V.; Agnandji, S.T.; Lell, B.; Yaro, S.; Yang, J.S.; Hoinard, D.; Weaver, S.C.; Vanhomwegen, J.; Salje, H.; et al. Seroepidemiological Reconstruction of Long-term Chikungunya Virus Circulation in Burkina Faso and Gabon. *J. Infect. Dis.* **2023**, *227*, 261–267. [CrossRef]
28. Ansumana, R.; Jacobsen, K.H.; Leski, T.A.; Covington, A.L.; Bangura, U.; Hodges, M.H.; Lin, B.; Bockarie, A.S.; Lamin, J.M.; Bockarie, M.J.; et al. Reemergence of chikungunya virus in Bo, Sierra Leone. *Emerg. Infect. Dis.* **2013**, *19*, 1108–1110. [CrossRef] [PubMed]
29. Agboli, E.; Zahouli, J.B.Z.; Badolo, A.; Jost, H. Mosquito-Associated Viruses and Their Related Mosquitoes in West Africa. *Viruses* **2021**, *13*, 891. [CrossRef]
30. Schoepp, R.J.; Rossi, C.A.; Khan, S.H.; Goba, A.; Fair, J.N. Undiagnosed acute viral febrile illnesses, Sierra Leone. *Emerg. Infect. Dis.* **2014**, *20*, 1176–1182. [CrossRef]
31. Dariano, D.F.; Taitt, C.R.; Jacobsen, K.H.; Bangura, U.; Bockarie, A.S.; Bockarie, M.J.; Lahai, J.; Lamin, J.M.; Leski, T.A.; Yasuda, C.; et al. Surveillance of Vector-Borne Infections (Chikungunya, Dengue, and Malaria) in Bo, Sierra Leone, 2012–2013. *Am. J. Trop. Med. Hyg.* **2017**, *97*, 1151–1154. [CrossRef] [PubMed]
32. Woodruff, A.W.; Bowen, E.T.; Platt, G.S. Viral infections in travellers from tropical Africa. *Br. Med. J.* **1978**, *1*, 956–958. [CrossRef]
33. Jentes, E.S.; Robinson, J.; Johnson, B.W.; Conde, I.; Sakouvougui, Y.; Iverson, J.; Beecher, S.; Bah, M.A.; Diakite, F.; Coulibaly, M.; et al. Acute arboviral infections in Guinea, West Africa, 2006. *Am. J. Trop. Med. Hyg.* **2010**, *83*, 388–394. [CrossRef]
34. Bane, S.; Rosenke, K.; Feldmann, F.; Meade-White, K.; Diawara, S.; Keita, M.; Maiga, O.; Diakite, M.; Safronetz, D.; Doumbia, S.; et al. Seroprevalence of Arboviruses in a Malaria Hyperendemic Area in Southern Mali. *Am. J. Trop. Med. Hyg.* **2024**, *111*, 107–112. [CrossRef]
35. Sow, A.; Nikolay, B.; Faye, O.; Cauchemez, S.; Cano, J.; Diallo, M.; Faye, O.; Sadio, B.; Ndiaye, O.; Weaver, S.C.; et al. Changes in the Transmission Dynamic of Chikungunya Virus in Southeastern Senegal. *Viruses* **2020**, *12*, 196. [CrossRef]
36. Tonto, P.B.; Sy, M.; Ndiaye, I.M.; Toure, M.; Gaye, A.; Aidara, M.; Mbaye, A.M.; Dia, A.K.; Diallo, M.A.; Gomis, J.F.; et al. Seroprevalence of chikungunya and o'nyong-nyong viruses in Senegal, West Africa. *medRxiv* **2024**. [CrossRef]
37. Nanfack Minkeu, F.; Vernick, K.D. A Systematic Review of the Natural Virome of Anopheles Mosquitoes. *Viruses* **2018**, *10*, 222. [CrossRef] [PubMed]
38. Posey, D.L.; O'Rourke, T.; Roehrig, J.T.; Lanciotti, R.S.; Weinberg, M.; Maloney, S. O'Nyong-nyong fever in West Africa. *Am. J. Trop. Med. Hyg.* **2005**, *73*, 32.
39. Safronetz, D.; Sacko, M.; Sogoba, N.; Rosenke, K.; Martellaro, C.; Traore, S.; Cisse, I.; Maiga, O.; Boisen, M.; Nelson, D.; et al. Vectorborne Infections, Mali. *Emerg. Infect. Dis.* **2016**, *22*, 340–342. [CrossRef] [PubMed]

40. Boisen, M.L.; Schieffelin, J.S.; Goba, A.; Oottamasathien, D.; Jones, A.B.; Shaffer, J.G.; Hastie, K.M.; Hartnett, J.N.; Momoh, M.; Fullah, M.; et al. Multiple circulating infections can mimic the early stages of viral hemorrhagic fevers and possible human exposure to filoviruses in Sierra Leone prior to the 2014 outbreak. *Viral Immunol.* **2015**, *28*, 19–31. [CrossRef]
41. Diarra, I.; Nurtop, E.; Sangare, A.K.; Sagara, I.; Pastorino, B.; Sacko, S.; Zeguime, A.; Coulibaly, D.; Fofana, B.; Gallian, P.; et al. Zika Virus Circulation in Mali. *Emerg. Infect. Dis.* **2020**, *26*, 945–952. [CrossRef]
42. Bayandin, R.B.; Makenov, M.T.; Boumbaly, S.; Stukolova, O.A.; Gladysheva, A.V.; Shipovalov, A.V.; Skarnovich, M.O.; Camara, O.; Toure, A.H.; Svyatchenko, V.A.; et al. The First Case of Zika Virus Disease in Guinea: Description, Virus Isolation, Sequencing, and Seroprevalence in Local Population. *Viruses* **2023**, *15*, 1620. [CrossRef]
43. Sene, O.; Sagne, S.N.; Bob, N.S.; Mhamadi, M.; Dieng, I.; Gaye, A.; Ba, H.; Dia, M.; Faye, E.T.; Diop, S.M.; et al. Re-Emergence of Rift Valley Fever Virus Lineage H in Senegal in 2022: In Vitro Characterization and Impact on Its Global Emergence in West Africa. *Viruses* **2024**, *16*, 1018. [CrossRef]
44. Ba, Y.; Sall, A.A.; Diallo, D.; Mondo, M.; Girault, L.; Dia, I.; Diallo, M. Re-emergence of Rift Valley fever virus in Barkedji (Senegal, West Africa) in 2002–2003: Identification of new vectors and epidemiological implications. *J. Am. Mosq. Control Assoc.* **2012**, *28*, 170–178. [CrossRef]
45. Troupin, C.; Ellis, I.; Doukoure, B.; Camara, A.; Keita, M.; Kagbadouno, M.; Bart, J.M.; Diallo, R.; Lacote, S.; Marianneau, P.; et al. Seroprevalence of brucellosis, Q fever and Rift Valley fever in domestic ruminants in Guinea in 2017–2019. *BMC Vet. Res.* **2022**, *18*, 64. [CrossRef]
46. Kanoute, Y.B.; Gragnon, B.G.; Schindler, C.; Bonfoh, B.; Schelling, E. Epidemiology of brucellosis, Q Fever and Rift Valley Fever at the human and livestock interface in northern Cote d'Ivoire. *Acta Trop.* **2017**, *165*, 66–75. [CrossRef] [PubMed]
47. Favier, C.; Chalvet-Monfray, K.; Sabatier, P.; Lancelot, R.; Fontenille, D.; Dubois, M.A. Rift Valley fever in West Africa: The role of space in endemicity. *Trop. Med. Int. Health* **2006**, *11*, 1878–1888. [CrossRef]
48. Clark, M.H.A.; Warimwe, G.M.; Di Nardo, A.; Lyons, N.A.; Gubbins, S. Systematic literature review of Rift Valley fever virus seroprevalence in livestock, wildlife and humans in Africa from 1968 to 2016. *PLoS Negl. Trop. Dis.* **2018**, *12*, e0006627. [CrossRef]
49. Ebogo-Belobo, J.T.; Kenmoe, S.; Abanda, N.N.; Bowo-Ngandji, A.; Mbaga, D.S.; Magoudjou-Pekam, J.N.; Kame-Ngasse, G.I.; Tchatchouang, S.; Menkem, E.Z.; Okobalemba, E.A.; et al. Contemporary epidemiological data of Rift Valley fever virus in humans, mosquitoes and other animal species in Africa: A systematic review and meta-analysis. *Vet. Med. Sci.* **2023**, *9*, 2309–2328. [CrossRef] [PubMed]
50. Durand, J.P.; Vallee, L.; de Pina, J.J.; Tolou, H. Isolation of a dengue type 1 virus from a soldier in West Africa (Cote d'Ivoire). *Emerg. Infect. Dis.* **2000**, *6*, 83–84. [CrossRef]
51. Saluzzo, J.F.; Cornet, M.; Castagnet, P.; Rey, C.; Digoutte, J.P. Isolation of dengue 2 and dengue 4 viruses from patients in Senegal. *Trans. R. Soc. Trop. Med. Hyg.* **1986**, *80*, 5. [CrossRef]
52. Bonney, J.H.K.; Pratt, D.; Ofori, M.; Hayashi, T.; Abankwa, A.; Awuku-Larbi, Y.; Kumordjie, S.; Agbodzi, B.; Salisu, M.; Mante, A.A.O.; et al. Molecular detection of dengue virus from febrile patients in Ghana. *BMC Infect. Dis.* **2024**, *24*, 1382. [CrossRef]
53. Bonney, J.H.K.; Hayashi, T.; Dadzie, S.; Agbosu, E.; Pratt, D.; Nyarko, S.; Asiedu-Bekoe, F.; Ido, E.; Sarkodie, B.; Ohta, N.; et al. Molecular detection of dengue virus in patients suspected of Ebola virus disease in Ghana. *PLoS ONE* **2018**, *13*, e0208907. [CrossRef]
54. Dieng, I.; Diagne, M.M.; Ndione, M.H.D.; Hedible, B.G.; Diop, M.; Adjoguoua, E.V.; Sylla, Y.; Kadjo, H.; Loucoubar, C.; Sall, A.A.; et al. Dengue virus serotype 2 imported case from Cote d'Ivoire to Senegal, 2017. *Transbound. Emerg. Dis.* **2022**, *69*, 3035–3040. [CrossRef]
55. L'Azou, M.; Succo, T.; Kamagate, M.; Ouattara, A.; Gilbernair, E.; Adjogoua, E.; Luxemburger, C. Dengue: Etiology of acute febrile illness in Abidjan, Cote d'Ivoire, in 2011–2012. *Trans. R. Soc. Trop. Med. Hyg.* **2015**, *109*, 717–722. [CrossRef]
56. Ouattara, C.A.; Traore, S.; Sangare, I.; Traore, T.I.; Meda, Z.C.; Savadogo, L.G.B. Spatiotemporal analysis of dengue fever in Burkina Faso from 2016 to 2019. *BMC Public Health* **2022**, *22*, 462. [CrossRef]
57. de Araujo Lobo, J.M.; Mores, C.N.; Bausch, D.G.; Christofferson, R.C. Short Report: Serological Evidence of Under-Reported Dengue Circulation in Sierra Leone. *PLoS Negl. Trop. Dis.* **2016**, *10*, e0004613. [CrossRef]
58. Manu, S.K.; Bonney, J.H.K.; Pratt, D.; Abdulai, F.N.; Agbosu, E.E.; Frimpong, P.O.; Adiku, T.K. Arbovirus circulation among febrile patients at the greater Accra Regional Hospital, Ghana. *BMC Res. Notes* **2019**, *12*, 332. [CrossRef]
59. de Brito Arduino, M.; Mucci, L.F.; Serpa, L.L.; Rodrigues Mde, M. Effect of salinity on the behavior of *Aedes aegypti* populations from the coast and plateau of southeastern Brazil. *J. Vector Borne Dis.* **2015**, *52*, 79–87. [CrossRef] [PubMed]
60. Whitehorn, J.; Kien, D.T.; Nguyen, N.M.; Nguyen, H.L.; Kyrylos, P.P.; Carrington, L.B.; Tran, C.N.; Quyen, N.T.; Thi, L.V.; Le Thi, D.; et al. Comparative Susceptibility of *Aedes albopictus* and *Aedes aegypti* to Dengue Virus Infection After Feeding on Blood of Viremic Humans: Implications for Public Health. *J. Infect. Dis.* **2015**, *212*, 1182–1190. [CrossRef]
61. Wichgers Schreur, P.J.; Vloet, R.P.M.; Kant, J.; van Keulen, L.; Gonzales, J.L.; Visser, T.M.; Koenraadt, C.J.M.; Vogels, C.B.F.; Kortekaas, J. Reproducing the Rift Valley fever virus mosquito-lamb-mosquito transmission cycle. *Sci. Rep.* **2021**, *11*, 1477. [CrossRef] [PubMed]

62. Turell, M.J.; Linthicum, K.J.; Patrican, L.A.; Davies, F.G.; Kairo, A.; Bailey, C.L. Vector competence of selected African mosquito (Diptera: Culicidae) species for Rift Valley fever virus. *J. Med. Entomol.* **2008**, *45*, 102–108. [CrossRef] [PubMed]
63. Wilke, A.B.B.; Vasquez, C.; Carvajal, A.; Moreno, M.; Fuller, D.O.; Cardenas, G.; Petrie, W.D.; Beier, J.C. Urbanization favors the proliferation of Aedes aegypti and Culex quinquefasciatus in urban areas of Miami-Dade County, Florida. *Sci. Rep.* **2021**, *11*, 22989. [CrossRef]
64. Tsetsarkin, K.A.; Vanlandingham, D.L.; McGee, C.E.; Higgs, S. A single mutation in chikungunya virus affects vector specificity and epidemic potential. *PLoS Pathog.* **2007**, *3*, e201. [CrossRef]
65. Kamgang, B.; Wilson-Bahun, T.A.; Irving, H.; Kusimo, M.O.; Lenga, A.; Wondji, C.S. Geographical distribution of Aedes aegypti and *Aedes albopictus* (Diptera: Culicidae) and genetic diversity of invading population of Ae. albopictus in the Republic of the Congo. *Wellcome Open Res.* **2018**, *3*, 79. [CrossRef]
66. Guindo-Coulibaly, N.; Adja, A.M.; Coulibaly, J.T.; Kpan, M.D.S.; Adou, K.A.; Zoh, D.D. Expansion of Aedes africanus (Diptera: Culicidae), a sylvatic vector of arboviruses, into an urban environment of Abidjan, Cote d'Ivoire. *J. Vector Ecol.* **2019**, *44*, 248–255. [CrossRef] [PubMed]
67. Ciota, A.T. West Nile virus and its vectors. *Curr. Opin. Insect Sci.* **2017**, *22*, 28–36. [CrossRef] [PubMed]
68. Haun, B.K.; Kamara, V.; Dweh, A.S.; Garalde-Machida, K.; Forkay, S.S.E.; Takaaze, M.; Namekar, M.; Wong, T.A.S.; Bell-Gam Woto, A.E.R.; Humphreys, P.; et al. Serological evidence of Ebola virus exposure in dogs from affected communities in Liberia: A preliminary report. *PLoS Negl. Trop. Dis.* **2019**, *13*, e0007614. [CrossRef] [PubMed]

Tropical Medicine and Infectious Disease

MDPI

Systematic Review

Chikungunya Fever and Rheumatoid Arthritis: A Systematic Review and Meta-Analysis

José Kennedy Amaral [1,*], Robert Taylor Schoen [2], Michael E. Weinblatt [3] and Estelita Lima Cândido [1]

[1] Postgraduate Program in Health Sciences, Faculty of Medicine, Federal University of Cariri, 284 Divino Salvador Street, Barbalha 63090-000, Ceará, Brazil; estelita.lima@ufca.edu.br
[2] Section of Rheumatology, Allergy, and Immunology, Yale University School of Medicine, 15 York Street, New Haven, CT 06510, USA; robert.schoen@yale.edu
[3] Division of Rheumatology, Inflammation and Immunity, Harvard Medical School, Brigham and Women's Hospital, 60 Fenwood Road, Boston, MA 02115, USA; mweinblatt@bwh.harvard.edu
* Correspondence: jkennedy-@hotmail.com

Abstract: Chikungunya fever (CHIKF) is a re-emerging infectious disease caused by the chikungunya virus (CHIKV), transmitted primarily by Aedes mosquitoes. A significant number progress to chronic chikungunya arthritis, which shares similarities with rheumatoid arthritis (RA). Despite evidence of a link between CHIKV infection and subsequent RA development, a comprehensive analysis of the relationship between these two diseases is lacking. This study systematically analyzes the incidence of RA after CHIKV infection and its immunological mechanisms, following PRISMA guidelines with literature searches across multiple databases up to 3 September 2024. Eligible studies included retrospective and prospective designs reporting RA diagnoses after CHIKV infection. Data extraction was performed independently, and the risk of bias was assessed using appropriate tools. Sixteen studies involving 2879 patients were included, with 449 individuals diagnosed with RA following CHIKV infection, resulting in a combined incidence of 13.7% (95% CI: 6.12% to 27.87%). High heterogeneity between studies was observed (I^2 = 96%), indicating variability related to diagnostic criteria and population characteristics. This review highlights the significant RA incidence after CHIKV infection, emphasizing the need for research on autoimmune mechanisms, long-term rheumatological follow-up, early diagnostic biomarkers, and CHIKV's long-term health impacts.

Keywords: chickungunya fever; rheumatoid arthritis; joint disease; autoimmune arthritis

1. Introduction

Chikungunya fever (CHIKF) is a mosquito-borne, viral infection that has re-emerged in global outbreaks over the past 75 years. First reported in 1952, CHIKF has since spread to over 100 countries, with over 4 million cases reported, particularly after the first case in the Americas in 2013 [1,2]. The chikungunya virus (CHIKV), a positive-sense single-stranded RNA *Alphavirus* virus is transmitted by *Aedes mosquitoes* (*Ae. aegypti* and *Ae. albopictus*) [3]. The disease presents with sudden fever, incapacitating polyarthritis, myalgia, rash, headache, and gastrointestinal symptoms, typically 2 to 6 days after infection [4]. While usually self-limiting, with recovery in 10 days, up to 40% of cases progress to a chronic phase, chronic chikungunya arthritis (CCA), characterized by persistent or deforming arthritis [5].

Following the global spread from Africa of the vectors of CHIKV, *A. aegypti* and *A. albopictus*, and the increase in international travel, there has been rapid geographic expansion of CHIKV infection. With the resultant increasing CCA cases, better characterization of the clinical features of CCA has been possible [6,7]. Within the clinical spectrum of CCA, some patients present as RA "mimics" with symmetric polyarthritis, morning stiffness, frequent hand involvement, and in some individuals, positive RA biomarkers. [8–10]. Not infrequently, these individuals meet ACR (American College of Rheumatology)/EULAR (European Alliance of Associations for Rheumatology) classification criteria for RA [11,12] Whether CCA mimics RA or whether CHIKV infection increases the risk of developing ongoing RA is still a subject of debate.

The similarities between CCA and RA are pathological as well as clinical [5,10,11,13]. RA is a systemic inflammatory disease of multifactorial etiology characterized by chronic and progressive synovitis [9–11]. RA pathogenesis involves interactions between genetic, environmental, and immunological factors, resulting in dysregulated immune responses and chronic inflammation, damaging joints and other organs [10]. Immunophenotyping of peripheral blood mononuclear cells in RA and CCA reveals a common inflammatory profile, suggesting shared immunological mechanisms. Viral persistence in joints, detection of viral genetic material in the synovium, and activation of innate and adaptive immune responses are mechanisms proposed to explain CCA pathogenesis. Autoimmunity induced by molecular mimicry or virus-induced tissue damage has also been considered [8,11].

There has long been interest in whether RA is linked to viral infection [12]. For CCA, there is a fundamental pathogenic question as to whether the arthritis phase results from persistent viral infection or a post-viral inflammatory process [13,14]. There is also a question as to whether CCA patients benefit from a disease-modifying treatment strategy, borrowed from the treatment of RA [11]. For these multiple reasons, we conducted a systematic review and meta-analysis to evaluate current evidence on the development of RA following CHIKV infection. We believe that the increasingly available data justify further investigation of pathogenic similarities between these two diseases and support CCA therapeutic strategies informed by RA treatment.

2. Materials and Methods

The study protocol was registered in the International Prospective Register of Systematic Reviews (PROSPERO) (protocol CRD42024585798). This study was conducted according to the Preferred Reporting Items for Systematic Reviews and Meta-Analyses (PRISMA) [15] guidelines to address the following question: "What are the characteristics and incidence of rheumatoid arthritis development in patients after chikungunya virus infection?"

2.1. *Information Sources*

We systematically searched PubMed, Cochrane Library, Scielo, LILACS, Web of Science, and Scopus for relevant literature published until 3 September 2024. We also incorporated studies found through manual searches using Google Scholar, gray literature, and reference lists. Articles in English, Spanish, or Portuguese were included.

2.2. *Eligibility Criteria*

Retrospective and prospective studies, randomized controlled trials, and case series reporting diagnosis of RA after CHIKV infection, with clinically and laboratory-confirmed testing for anti-CHIKV-specific immunoglobulin M (for acute cases) or immunoglobulin G (post-exposure) detected by enzyme-linked immunosorbent assay (ELISA) or RNA virus by reverse-transcriptase polymerase chain reaction were included. Studies were excluded if they did not include laboratory confirmation of CHIKV, did not follow the ACR-EULAR classification criteria, or presented insufficient data for analysis. We excluded from this systematic review: letters to the editor, editorials, review articles, commentaries, preclinical trials, and papers without relevant data.

2.3. Search Strategy

Search terms included combinations of free-text and MeSH or Emtree terms for CHIK and RA, including ("Chikungunya virus" (MeSH) OR "Chikungunya fever" (MeSH) OR "CHIKV" OR "Chikungunya infection" OR "Chikungunya" OR "CHIK" OR "CHIKV") AND ("Arthritis, Rheumatoid" (MeSH) OR "Rheumatoid arthritis" OR "Autoimmune arthritis" OR "RA"). Information about the databases used, search dates, search methods, and the number of studies retrieved is provided in the Supplementary Materials (Table S1).

2.4. Selection Process

Two independent reviewers (J.K.A. and R.T.S.) screened titles and abstracts based on the eligibility criteria. Studies with uncertain relevance were included to ensure all potentially relevant work was considered. Disagreements were resolved through discussion, with a third reviewer involved if necessary. The same process was applied to full-text reviews, with further evaluation of studies with unclear relevance at the abstract stage.

2.5. Data Collection Process

Independent reviewers (J.K.A. and R.T.S.) extracted data using a standardized form (Table S2). Afterward, a second reviewer independently verified the data to ensure all relevant information was included. Any discrepancies were resolved through discussion, with a third reviewer involved if necessary. The form captured details such as author, publication year, country, study design, patient demographics, type of chikungunya diagnosis, number of RA cases, comparators, evaluation measures, symptoms, clinical progression, and study results.

2.6. Data Items

Data were collected on the following outcomes: the incidence of RA, defined by the percentage of patients who developed RA after CHIKV infection, as diagnosed by the authors of the included studies using standard clinical and laboratory criteria; the clinical and demographic characteristics of patients, including mean age (±standard deviation), sex (male/female), country of origin, and type of chikungunya diagnosis (acute or post-exposure), as determined by the detection of anti-CHIKV IgM or IgG antibodies or viral RNA by PCR; the measures used to assess RA, such as clinical examinations, laboratory tests, and established diagnostic criteria; the clinical evolution of patients, including descriptions of symptoms, duration of arthritis, clinical progression of the disease, and response to specific treatments, when applicable; and other relevant outcomes, including any other relevant findings associated with the development of RA following CHIK infection, as reported in the included studies.

2.7. Study Risk of Bias Assessment

The risk of bias in the included studies was assessed using tools appropriate to each study design, focusing on those that confirmed CHIKV infection through serological tests (IgM/IgG anti-CHIKV) or other validated methods. Two reviewers independently evaluated the risk of bias using the Newcastle–Ottawa Scale (NOS) for cohort studies, the Joanna Briggs Institute (JBI) Critical Appraisal Checklist for case series and observational studies, and the RoB 2.0 tool for randomized controlled trials [16–19].

3. Results

3.1. Study Selection

A total of 4392 studies were retrieved from the database searches. After exclusion by reading the titles and/or abstracts and duplicates, only 46 articles were selected for full reading. Sixteen studies met the eligibility criteria and were included in the systematic review (Figure 1).

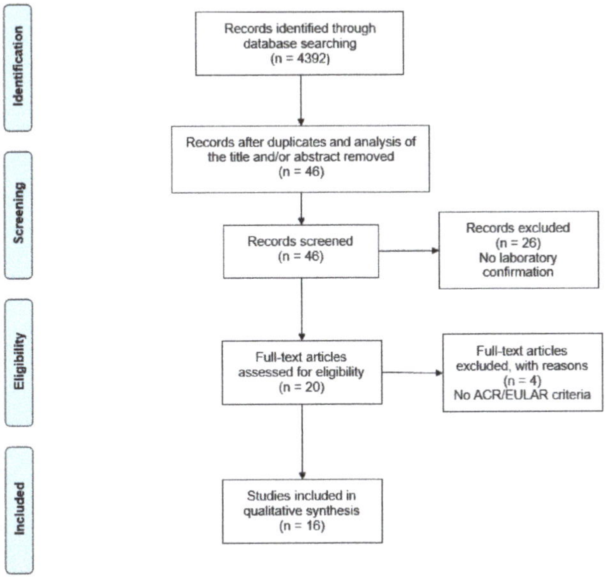

Figure 1. PRISMA flow diagram of search results. PRISMA: Preferred Reporting Items for Systematic Reviews and Meta-Analyses.

3.2. Study Characteristics

The studies included in this systematic review were conducted in diverse geographical and epidemiological settings, reflecting the wide geographic distribution of CHIKV infection and its rheumatological consequences. Two cross-sectional studies were conducted in Brazil [20] and Colombia [21]. Nine cohort studies included research from Bangladesh [22], the United States [23], France [24], India [25–27], Colombia [28,29], and Reunion Island [30]. Four case series studies were conducted in the United States [31], France [32], Reunion Island [33], and Brazil [34]. The randomized controlled trial was conducted in India [35].

3.3. Risk of Bias in Studies

3.3.1. Cross-Sectional and Case Series Studies

Among the cross-sectional studies, both Hayd et al. [20] and Tritsch et al. [21] were rated as having a moderate risk of bias. These studies showed limitations in controlling for potential confounding factors that could affect the validity of their findings. Similarly, among the case series studies, there was variable bias risk. While some case series, such as Javelle et al. [33], were rated with low risk of bias due to their clear inclusion criteria and consistent measurement of outcomes, others, including Miner et al. [31], Bouquillard and Combe [32], and Amaral et al. [34], were assessed as having a moderate risk of bias due to concerns related to participant selection and the handling of incomplete data.

3.3.2. Cohort Studies

A significant proportion of the cohort studies (n = 7 of 9) were rated with low risk of bias. These studies, such as Pollett et al. [23], Manimunda et al. [25], Segura-Charry et al. [28], Rodriguez-Morales et al. [29], Paul et al. [26], Mathew et al. [27], and Guillot et al. [30], adhered to rigorous methodological standards, including valid and reliable measurement of exposures and outcomes, identification and control of confounding factors, and sufficient follow-up duration to capture relevant outcomes.

Two cohort studies were rated with a moderate risk of bias. Hossain et al. [22] and Bouquillard et al. [24] had incomplete follow-up and inadequate handling of confounding factors that could introduce bias into their findings.

3.3.3. Randomized Controlled Trials

The randomized controlled trial by Ravindran and Alias [35] was rated with some bias concerns using the RoB 2.0 tool. The study was an open-label design, raising potential bias in the measurement of subjective outcomes. Although the trial demonstrated strength in areas like randomization and handling of missing data, the open-label nature could have influenced participant behavior or reporting, leading to "some concerns" about the overall risk of bias.

The details are reported in the Supplementary Materials.

3.4. Results of Individual Studies

A total of 2879 patients infected by CHIKV were found in the included studies, with 449 diagnosed with RA. The studies differed by location and methods but consistently identified patients meeting RA diagnostic criteria after infection. Common symptoms included persistent joint pain, morning stiffness, polyarthralgia, joint swelling, and autoantibodies such as rheumatoid factor (RF) and anti-cyclic citrullinated peptide (anti-CCP). Severe cases showed bone erosions, synovitis, and required advanced therapies like tumor necrosis factor (TNF) blockers and other biologics.

For example, Segura-Charry et al. [28] reported that 87 of 410 patients developed RA, with many requiring biologics therapy due to disease severity. In Guillot et al. [30], 40 of 159 patients had persistent symptoms up to 13 years post infection, highlighting the chronic nature of RA after CHIKV. Bouquillard and Combe [32] and Javelle et al. [33] demonstrated the effectiveness of methotrexate (MTX) in alleviating symptoms and slowing disease progression. Ravindran and Alias found combination therapy with MTX, sulfasalazine, and hydroxychloroquine (HCQ) more effective than HCQ monotherapy in reducing RA activity after CHIKV [35].

See Table 1 for details on each study, including diagnosed cases and clinical characteristics.

Table 1. Characteristics and outcomes of studies evaluating rheumatoid arthritis following chikungunya virus infection.

Author, Year and Country	Study Design	N° Patients, N° Male/FemaleAge Mean ± SD or Median (Years)	Chikungunya Diagnosis Type	N° Rheumatoid Arthritis Diagnosed Patients	Comparators	Evaluation Measure	Description of Symptoms and Clinical Evolution	Results	Risk of Bias
Hayd et al., 2020 [20], Brazil	Cross-sectional analysis	160 patients: 40 with chronic arthritis (CHIKV), 40 without arthritis (CHIKV exposed), 40 with RA (controls), 40 healthy controls; Predominantly female; Age: 48.6 ± 11.5 (CHIKV arthritis), 43.9 ± 16.3 (CHIKV without arthritis), 51 ± 13.4 (RA Controls), 31.9 ± 11.7 (Healthy controls)	RT-qPCR confirmed CHIKV cases	4 patients	Rheumatoid arthritis controls, CHIKV exposed without arthritis, healthy controls	DAS28, EQ-5D-5L, MSQ	Initial symptoms: fever, joint pain, headache, myalgia. Chronic symptoms included persistent arthritis affecting fingers, knees, wrists, toes, and ankles, with some patients experiencing relapsing-remitting joint pain.	Over 2 years post-infection, moderate arthritis severity was reported, significantly affecting the quality of life due to pain	Moderate [a]
Hossain et al., 2022 [22], Bangladesh	Retrospective observa-tional cohort study	143 patients: 73 male/70 female, age: 43.3 ± 11.5	RT-PCR or IgM/IgG positive	7 patients	Patients with pre-existing arthritis (RA, SpA, OA), patients without arthritis	HAQ, RF, ACPA, X-ray sacroiliac joint, Ultrasound (musculoskeletal)	Initial symptoms included fever, polyarthralgia, symmetrical joint involvement; chronic phase symptoms included persistent mono/oligoarthritis, polyarthritis, RA, SpA.	At 1-year follow-up, 41.9% of patients had post-chikungunya chronic inflammatory rheumatism (pCHIK-CIR). Risk factors included female gender, positive IgG, and moderate to severe functional disability.	Moderate [b]
Miner et al., 2015 [31], USA	Retrospective case series	10 patients: 3 Male/7 Female, Age range: 18–57 years	Positive for anti-CHIKV IgG (ELISA)	8 patients	none	Complete blood count, comprehensive metabolic panel, ESR, CRP, CCP, RF, ANA, CyTOF analysis of PBMCs	Acute symptoms: fever, rash, headache, symmetric polyarthritis. Chronic symptoms: persistent arthritis (hands, feet, ankles), morning stiffness, pain, joint swelling	8 of 10 patients developed RA; immune profile (T cells, NK cells) was similar to RA, highlighting diagnostic challenges.	Moderate [c]
Tritsch et al., 2020 [21], Colombia	Cross-sectional follow-up	120 patients: 17 Male/103 Female, Age Mean: 51 ± 14 years	Clinically confirmed CHIKV, serologically confirmed (IgM and IgG)	2 patients	none	EQ-5D questionnaire, joint count, global pain score	54% of patients reported persistent joint pain 40 months post-infection; most common type of pain was relapsing-remitting; stiffness was reported by 75% of patients post-immobility.	Around 1 in 8 patients had persistent joint pain 3 years after infection. Over half of patients with joint pain experienced relapsing-remitting symptoms.	Moderate [a]

Table 1. *Cont.*

Author, Year and Country	Study Design	N° Patients, N° Male/FemaleAge Mean ± SD or Median (Years)	Chikungunya Diagnosis Type	N° Rheumatoid Arthritis Diagnosed Patients	Comparators	Evaluation Measure	Description of Symptoms and Clinical Evolution	Results	Risk of Bias
Pollett et al., 2023 [23], USA	Retrospective cohort study	195 patients: 103 Male/92 Female; Median age: 42 years [IQR 31–54]	Diagnosed using RT-PCR or serological testing (IgM/IgG)	7 patients	Matched non-CHIKV controls (1:4 ratio) based on age, gender, beneficiary status, and healthcare encounter date	Incident rheumatic diagnoses, healthcare utilization, conditional logistic regression models	Acute symptoms included fever, polyarthralgia, backache, headache, fatigue; post-CHIKV rheumatological sequelae such as arthralgia, polyarthritis, polymyalgia rheumatica, and RA were observed.	CHIKV infection was associated with a significantly higher risk of developing rheumatological sequelae (aOR = 1.911, $p = 0.002$). 32.3% of CHIKV cases had incident rheumatic diagnoses compared to 20.0% of controls. No significant demographic, clinical, or occupational predictors were identified for rheumatic complications.	Low [b]
Bouquillard et al., 2017 [24], France	Prospective observational cohort study	307 patients: 52 male/255 female; Mean age: 54 ± 12.6 years (24–87)	Serology (IgM and/or IgG positive)	13 patients	Patients with serological confirmation vs. clinical diagnosis; evolution of symptoms under different treatments.	HAQ score, VAS pain, synovial fluid analysis	Chronic joint pain persisted in 83.1% of patients after 32 months; synovitis observed in 64.2%, primarily affecting wrists, fingers, and ankles. Symptoms included fever, arthralgia, swollen joints, myalgia, rash, headache.	83.1% of patients reported persistent joint pain; 4% developed RA post-infection; significant functional impairment was moderate, with a mean HAQ score of 0.44 ± 0.5.	Moderate [b]
Bouquillard and Combe, 2009 [32], France	Prospective case series	21 patients: 13 female/8 male, Mean age: 57 ± 12 years	Serology confirmed (IgM and IgG antibodies)	21 patients	none	ESR, CRP, RF, anti-CCP, radiographs, MRI	Persistent arthritis from onset of CHIKV infection; 18 with symmetric polyarthritis, 3 with oligoarthritis; high ESR, positive RF in 57.1%, anti-CCP in 28.6%, erosions in hands/feet.	Severe outcomes in most cases; radiological evidence of joint damage in 80% of patients; 6 required TNF blockers due to inadequate response to methotrexate; suggests viral role in RA initiation.	Moderate [c]
Manimunda et al., 2010 [25], India	Prospective observational cohort study	203 patients: 96 Male/107 Female; Median age: 35 years [IQR 25–44]	Serologically confirmed (IgM antibody ELISA)	34 patients	None	ESR, X-ray, MRI, anti-CCP, RF	Acute symptoms: fever, joint pain, rash; chronic symptoms at 10 months: joint pain, swelling, fatigue; X-ray and MRI showed joint effusion, bony erosion, marrow edema, synovial thickening, tendinitis, tenosynovitis.	Chronic arthritis confirmed in 75% of patients at 10 months; 36% met ACR criteria for RA; joint erosion observed in some patients, proving that CHIK arthritis is chronic inflammatory erosive arthritis.	Low [b]

Table 1. *Cont.*

Author, Year and Country	Study Design	N° Patients, N° Male/FemaleAge Mean ± SD or Median (Years)	Chikungunya Diagnosis Type	N° Rheumatoid Arthritis Diagnosed Patients	Comparators	Evaluation Measure	Description of Symptoms and Clinical Evolution	Results	Risk of Bias
Segura-Charry et al., 2021 [28], Colombia	Retrospective observational longitudinal study	410 patients: 47 Male/363 Female; Mean age: 57.3 ± 11.7 years	Clinical and serological confirmation (IgG)	87 patients	none	Clinical assessment by expert rheumatologists, paraclinical tests (autoantibodies, acute phase reagents), imaging studies, use of ACR/EULAR and ASAS criteria	Persistent musculoskeletal and joint symptoms for more than 3 months, with 46.3% non-inflammatory arthralgias, 21.9% post-viral polyarthritis, 20.3% de novo RA	20.3% developed RA post-CHIKV, 58.6% seropositive for RA; significant need for advanced pharmacological measures, including biological therapy in some cases.	Low [b]
Javelle et al., 2015 [33], Reunion Island	Retrospective case series	159 patients: 40 male/119 female; Median age: 51 years (range 16–80)	Clinical and serological confirmation (RT-PCR, IgM, IgG)	40 patients	none	Time to first consultation, response to methotrexate (MTX), need for additional treatments	Persistent musculoskeletal pain, polyarthritis, spondyloarthritis; median delay of 2 years from infection to rheumatologist consultation; 66% had prolonged acute infection	MTX was effective in 75% of treated patients; hydroxychloroquine and ribavirin were ineffective; need for specific management guidelines to prevent progression to chronic disease.	Low [c]
Amaral et al., 2018 [34], Brazil	Retrospective case series	50 patients: 4 Male/46 Female; Mean age: 61.9 ± 12.5 years	Clinical and serological confirmation (IgG serology by ELISA)	11 patients	none	VAS, Swollen and Tender Joint Count	Chronic symptoms persisted for more than 12 weeks post-infection; polyarthralgia, polyarthritis, morning stiffness, and tenosynovitis reported in many patients.	Methotrexate significantly reduced pain and disease activity; rapid reduction in VAS pain scores from baseline to 4 and 8 weeks; well-tolerated with no serious adverse events.	Moderate [c]
Rodriguez-Morales et al., 2016 [36], Colombia	Retrospective observational cohort study	283 patients: 110 male (39%), 173 female (61%); Median age: 29 years (IQR 17–42)	Clinical confirmation and serological testing (IgM/IgG antibodies)	152 patients	None	Relative risk (RR), Kaplan-Meier survival curves, Cox regression	Persistent polyarthralgia (pCHIK-CPA) with symptoms including morning stiffness (49.5%), joint edema (40.6%), and joint redness (16.6%); higher prevalence of symptoms in patients > 40 years and females; significant persistence of symptoms up to 26 weeks.	53.7% of patients developed RA (pCHIK-CPA); more common in patients > 40 years old (69.7%) compared to ≤40 years old (47.8%); higher prevalence in females (59.5%) than males (44.5%); 19.4% of patients required ongoing medical care for persistent symptoms	Low [b]

Table 1. *Cont.*

Author, Year and Country	Study Design	N° Patients, N° Male/FemaleAge Mean ± SD or Median (Years)	Chikungunya Diagnosis Type	N° Rheumatoid Arthritis Diagnosed Patients	Comparators	Evaluation Measure	Description of Symptoms and Clinical Evolution	Results	Risk of Bias
Ravindran and Alias, 2016 [35], India	Randomized controlled open-label clinical trial	72 patients: 37 in combination therapy, 35 in monotherapy; Combination group: 4 male, 33 female; Monotherapy group: 5 male, 30 female; Age Mean ± SD: Combination: 54.05 ± 6.67, Monotherapy: 56.6 ± 7.64	Serologically confirmed (virus-specific IgM antibodies)	12 patients	Combination therapy (MTX, SSZ, and HCQ) vs. HCQ monotherapy	DAS28, HAQ, VAS	Persistent arthritis for >1 year post-CHIKV infection; symptoms included swollen joints, tenderness, and high disease activity. Both groups were previously on HCQ with active disease; assessed for response to combination therapy versus monotherapy.	Combination therapy significantly improved DAS28, HAQ, and VAS compared to monotherapy; 85% achieved EULAR good response in combination group vs. 14% in monotherapy group; combination therapy more effective in achieving low disease activity and reducing pain.	Some concerns [d]
Paul et al., 2011 [26], India	Prospective observa-tional cohort study	150 patients: 40 male/110 female; Age range: 20–60 years	Serological confirmation (IgM capture ELISA)	5 patients	None	Symptom duration, response to antimalarials and steroids	100% of patients had arthralgia, 78% had arthritis, 22% had persistent symptoms beyond one year; common symptoms included fever, rash, and morning stiffness; antimalarials and short courses of steroids were partially effective in some cases.	22% developed chronic symptoms; 5% of patients developed RA after CHIKV infection; RA cases had anti-CCP positivity; synovial biopsies showed chronic inflammation.	Low [b]
Mathew et al., 2011 [27], India	Retrospective observa-tional cohort study	437 patients: 124 male/313 female; Mean age: 48.37 ± 13.62 years	Clinical confirmation and serology (IgM antibodies)	6 patients	None	Pain site assessment, ACR criteria for rheumatic diseases, lab tests (ESR, CRP, RF, anti-CCP), musculoskeletal ultrasound	Common pain sites: knee (83.3%), ankle (63.2%), lower back (49.4%); 57% had post-viral polyarthralgia, 22% had post-viral polyarthritis.	8.3% incidence of RMSK pain in naïve group; higher prevalence of chronic rheumatic disorders post-CHIKV, including RA and seronegative spondyloarthritis.	Low [b]

Table 1. *Cont.*

Author, Year and Country	Study Design	N° Patients, N° Male/FemaleAge Mean ± SD or Median (Years)	Chikungunya Diagnosis Type	N° Rheumatoid Arthritis Diagnosed Patients	Comparators	Evaluation Measure	Description of Symptoms and Clinical Evolution	Results	Risk of Bias
Guillot et al., 2020 [30], Reunion Island	Retrospective observational cohort study	159 patients: Gender distribution not fully specified; Age data not provided	Clinical confirmation and serological testing (IgM/IgG antibodies)	40 patients	none	Clinical examination, autoantibodies (ACPA, RF, ANA), radiographic evaluations, DAS28 score, BASDAI score	Inflammatory joint symptoms persisted after 13 years; higher prevalence of positive autoantibodies (antinuclear or ACPA) without seroconversion, and radiographic joint damage in a subgroup	23.3% of patients initially diagnosed with CHIK-related inflammatory joint symptoms continued to have symptoms after 13 years; long-term IgM positivity and radiographic damage were more frequent in the persistence group.	Low [b]

ANA: antinuclear antibody; BASDAI: bath ankylosing spondylitis disease activity index; CCP: cyclic citrullinated peptide; CHIKV: chikungunya virus; CRP: C-reactive protein; CyTOF: cytometry by time-of-flight; DAS28: Disease Activity Score in 28 joints; EQ-5D-5L: The EuroQol 5-Dimension 5-level; ESR: erythrocyte sedimentation rate; HAQ: Health Assessment Questionnaire; MRI: magnetic resonance imaging; MSQ: musculoskeletal stiffness questionnaire; OA: osteoarthritis; PBMCs: peripheral blood mononuclear cells; RA: rheumatoid arthritis; RF: rheumatoid factor; RMSK: rheumatic-musculoskeletal; RT-qPCR: reverse transcription-quantitative (polymerase chain reaction); SpA: spondyloarthritis; TNF: tumor necrosis factor; VAS: visual analogue scale. [a]: Based on The Joanna Briggs Institute Critical Appraisal tool for cross-sectional analysis studies. [b]: Based on The Joanna Briggs Institute Critical Appraisal tool for cohort studies. [c]: Based on the Newcastle–Ottawa Scale (NOS) tool for case series. [d]: Based on RoB 2.0 tool for randomized trials.

3.5. Quality Assessment

Most of the studies included in the systematic review demonstrated good methodological quality, with low or moderate risk of bias. The rigorous application of the NOS, JBI, and RoB 2.0 bias assessment tools allowed for a clear identification of the strengths and limitations of each study.

3.6. Meta-Analysis

The combined proportion of patients who developed RA after CHIKV infection was 13.7% (IC 95%: 6.12% to 27.87%), based on the random effects model, due to high heterogeneity among studies ($I^2 = 96\%$, $Q = 373.00$, $p < 0.0001$). The graph in Figure 2 presents the individual estimates of RA proportion for each study, as well as the combined estimate obtained through the random effects model. After excluding cross-sectional studies and case series from the meta-analysis, heterogeneity reduced from 96% to 76.8% ($Q = 33.4969$, $p < 0.0001$), indicating better homogeneity among the remaining studies.

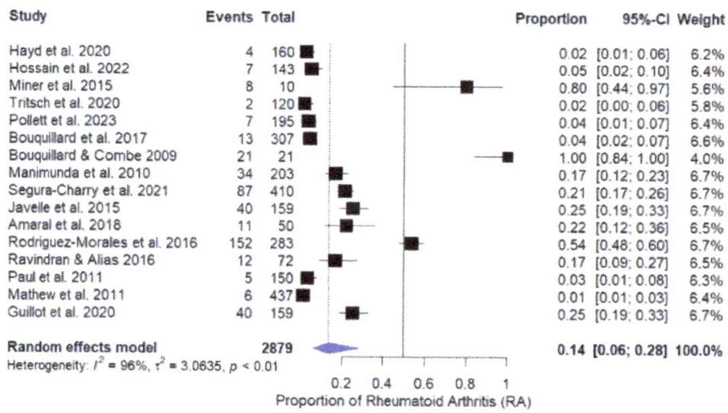

Figure 2. Forest plot of proportion of rheumatoid arthritis in patients after chikungunya infection [20–35].

The analysis only with cohort studies classified as having low risk of bias resulted in an incidence of rheumatoid arthritis of 17.7% (95% CI: 4.2–31.3%). Although heterogeneity decreased compared to the full meta-analysis, it still remained high ($I^2 = 81.07\%$).

The certainty of the evidence was assessed using the GRADE approach, considering risk of bias, inconsistency, imprecision, publication bias, and applicability of the results. For the incidence of RA post CHIKV, the certainty was considered moderate, downgraded due to inconsistency ($I^2 = 96\%$, IC 95%: 6.12–27.87%).

A forest plot showing the proportions of patients who developed rheumatoid arthritis after chikungunya infection in each study is included in the meta-analysis. The diamond at the bottom represents the combined proportion with a 95% confidence interval. The random effects model was used due to the high heterogeneity observed.

4. Discussion

This systematic review is, to our knowledge, the first to explore the relationship between CHIKV infection and the subsequent development of RA. Despite the heterogeneity of RA incidence among these studies, the meta-analysis suggests that a significant proportion of patients develop RA after CHIKV infection. However, the observed variability indicates that factors such as population characteristics, diagnostic methods, and follow-up duration may influence results. Our systematic review was restricted to studies that assessed RA as recognized in ACR-EULAR classification criteria [11]. Rodríguez-Morales et al. conducted a more general review in which they classified RA as part of a group called "post-CHIK chronic arthritis" that also included post-viral or nonspecific arthritis and seronegative spondylitis, finding a prevalence of 13.66%. However, they did not specifically evaluate RA separately [36].

Despite the variation in follow-up time among the studies in this review, we suggest that a longer period of time may be necessary to identify RA patients after CHIKV infection, as demonstrated in the study by Guillot et al. [30]. We acknowledge that the absence of a standardized observation period among the studies may have influenced the variability of the estimates, representing a limitation of this analysis.

Many CCA patients develop RA symptoms that clinically resemble classic RA, such as persistent joint pain, morning stiffness, polyarthralgia, and joint swelling [37–39]. But is this RA or an RA "mimic"? Many of these patients had severe disease, with joint erosions and synovitis, suggesting that CHIKV may cause the same inflammatory processes associated with RA, as described in another review [5]. The presence of auto-antibodies, such as RF and anti-CCP, also indicates that CHIKV may trigger autoimmunity, clinically indistinguishable from RA in non-CHIKV-infected individuals [8].

These clinical features are consistent with the known pathogenesis of post-CHIKV infection RA [14]. Viral persistence and molecular mimicry are possible mechanisms for the development of RA after CHIKV infection. Bouquillard et al. demonstrated that viral components can remain in synovial tissue long after acute infection, leading to chronic inflammation [32]. Additionally, Miner et al. [31] and Guillot et al. [30] report that CHIKV-induced arthritis shares immunological characteristics with idiopathic RA.

The efficacy of treatments for RA, such as MTX and biologic therapy in patients with CHIKV-induced arthritis has been documented in studies by Bouquillard and Combe [32] and Javelle et al. [33]. In these cohorts, patients with more severe manifestations required more aggressive treatment, such as TNF inhibitors, reflecting the chronic and refractory nature of post-CHIKV RA. These treatments significantly improved outcomes, reducing pain and disease activity. However, a recent clinical trial review did not demonstrate additional benefits of these drugs compared to anti-inflammatories or placebo [40].

Our review and meta-analysis included mostly observational studies, which may represent an important limitation because this type of study is more susceptible to selection bias and residual confounding. This may contribute to the high heterogeneity observed in the results (reduction of I^2 from 96% to 76.8%), and the incidence estimate, which went from 16.2% to 12.4%. However, due to the nature of the topic investigated, there is a limited availability of randomized controlled trials that could reduce these biases. Another limitation that should be mentioned is the variation in sample sizes (between 10 and 437 patients), which may influence the precision of the pooled estimates.

Future studies should prioritize the standardization of diagnostic criteria and the long-term follow-up of specific subgroups in order to more accurately clarify the risk factors for the development of RA after CHIKV infection. Moreover, research focused on early interventions is essential to reduce the impact of this disease. Given the chronic and debilitating nature of CHIKV-associated RA, it is crucial to explore the mechanisms of autoimmunity triggered by the virus. For this, longitudinal studies with well-defined cohorts are fundamental, allowing not only for a better understanding of disease progression but also for the identification of biomarkers that facilitate early diagnosis. Finally, clinical trials are indispensable to assess the long-term efficacy and safety of biological therapies and combined treatments, offering new perspectives for therapeutic management.

5. Conclusions

This systematic review and meta-analysis revealed that a significant proportion of patients infected with CHIKV develop RA, with a combined estimate of 13.7% (95% CI: 6.12% to 27.87%). However, the high heterogeneity between the studies (I^2 = 96%) indicates considerable variability in the findings, suggesting that factors such as differences in diagnostic criteria, study populations, and follow-up durations may have influenced the results.

These findings reinforce the need for long-term rheumatological follow-up in patients who have survived CHIKV infection, especially in endemic regions. The identification of autoimmune mechanisms associated with viral infection and the development of biomarkers for early diagnosis are important areas for future investigations.

Supplementary Materials: The following supporting information can be downloaded at: https://www.mdpi.com/article/10.3390/tropicalmed10020054/s1, Table S1: Details of risk of bias assessments based on the Newcastle–Ottawa Scale (NOS) for cohort studies; Table S2: Details of risk of bias assessments based on The Joanna Briggs Institute Critical Appraisal tool for cross-sectional analysis studies; Table S3: Details of risk of bias assessments based on The Joanna Briggs Institute Critical Appraisal tool for cohort studies; Table S4: Details of risk of bias assessments based on The Joanna Briggs Institute Critical Appraisal tool for case series; Table S5: Details of risk of bias assessments based on RoB 2.0 tool for randomized trials.

Author Contributions: Conceptualization, J.K.A.; methodology, J.K.A.; software, J.K.A.; validation, J.K.A., R.T.S., M.E.W. and E.L.C.; formal analysis, J.K.A.; investigation, J.K.A. and R.T.S.; resources, J.K.A. and M.E.W.; data curation, J.K.A.; writing—original draft preparation, J.K.A. and R.T.S.; writing—review and editing, J.K.A., R.T.S., M.E.W. and E.L.C.; visualization, J.K.A.; supervision, R.T.S. and E.L.C.; project administration, J.K.A. All authors have read and agreed to the published version of the manuscript.

Funding: This research received no external funding.

Data Availability Statement: The original contributions presented in this study are included in the article and Supplementary Materials. Further inquiries can be directed to the corresponding author.

Conflicts of Interest: The authors declare no conflicts of interest.

References

1. Costa, L.B.; Barreto, F.K.A.; Barreto, M.C.A.; dos Santos, T.H.P.; Andrade, M.d.M.O.d.; Farias, L.A.B.G.; de Freitas, A.R.R.; Martinez, M.J.; Cavalcanti, L.P.d.G. Epidemiology and Economic Burden of Chikungunya: A Systematic Literature Review. *Trop. Med. Infect. Dis.* **2023**, *8*, 301. [CrossRef]
2. Ferreira de Almeida, I.; Codeço, C.T.; Lana, R.M.; Bastos, L.S.; Oliveira, S.d.S.; Ferreira, D.A.d.C.; Godinho, V.B.; Riback, T.I.S.; Cruz, O.G.; Coelho, F.C. The Expansion of Chikungunya in Brazil. *Lancet Reg. Health Am.* **2023**, *25*, 100571. [CrossRef]
3. Bartholomeeusen, K.; Daniel, M.; LaBeaud, D.A.; Gasque, P.; Peeling, R.W.; Stephenson, K.E.; Ng, L.F.P.; Ariën, K.K. Chikungunya Fever. *Nat. Rev. Dis. Primers* **2023**, *9*, 17, Erratum in *Nat. Rev. Dis. Primers* **2023**, *9*, 26. [CrossRef] [PubMed]
4. Mourad, O.; Makhani, L.; Chen, L.H. Chikungunya: An Emerging Public Health Concern. *Curr. Infect. Dis. Rep.* **2022**, *24*, 217–228. [CrossRef]
5. Amaral, J.K.; Taylor, P.C.; Schoen, R.T. Bone Erosions and Joint Damage Caused by Chikungunya Virus: A Systematic Review. *Rev. Soc. Bras. Med. Trop.* **2024**, *57*, e00404. [CrossRef] [PubMed]
6. Wahid, B.; Ali, A.; Rafique, S.; Idrees, M. Global Expansion of Chikungunya Virus: Mapping the 64-Year History. *Int. J. Infect. Dis.* **2017**, *58*, 69–76. [CrossRef]
7. Charrel, R.N.; de Lamballerie, X.; Raoult, D. Chikungunya Outbreaks—The Globalization of Vector-Borne Diseases. *N. Engl. J. Med.* **2007**, *356*, 769–771. [CrossRef]
8. Bezerra, L.A.; da Silva Bastos, Y.C.; Gonçales, J.P.; Silva Júnior, J.V.J.; De Lorena, V.M.B.; Duarte, A.L.B.P.; Marques, C.D.L.; Coêlho, M.R.C.D. Synergism between Chikungunya Virus Infection and Rheumatoid Arthritis on Cytokine Levels: Clinical Implications? *Braz. J. Microbiol.* **2023**, *54*, 885–890. [CrossRef] [PubMed]

9. Alivernini, S.; Firestein, G.S.; McInnes, I.B. The Pathogenesis of Rheumatoid Arthritis. *Immunity* **2022**, *55*, 2255–2270. [CrossRef] [PubMed]
10. Scherer, H.U.; Häupl, T.; Burmester, G.R. The Etiology of Rheumatoid Arthritis. *J. Autoimmun.* **2020**, *110*, 102400. [CrossRef] [PubMed]
11. Aletaha, D.; Neogi, T.; Silman, A.J.; Funovits, J.; Felson, D.T.; Bingham, C.O., 3rd; Birnbaum, N.S.; Burmester, G.R.; Bykerk, V.P.; Cohen, M.D.; et al. 2010 Rheumatoid Arthritis Classification Criteria: An American College of Rheumatology/European League Against Rheumatism Collaborative Initiative. *Arthritis Rheum.* **2010**, *62*, 2569–2581. [CrossRef] [PubMed]
12. Amaral, J.K.; Bingham, C.O., 3rd; Taylor, P.C.; Vilá, L.M.; Weinblatt, M.E.; Schoen, R.T. Pathogenesis of Chronic Chikungunya Arthritis: Resemblances and Links with Rheumatoid Arthritis. *Travel Med. Infect. Dis.* **2023**, *52*, 102534. [CrossRef] [PubMed]
13. Kudaeva, F.M.; Speechley, M.R.; Pope, J.E. A Systematic Review of Viral Exposures as a Risk for Rheumatoid Arthritis. *Semin. Arthritis Rheum.* **2019**, *48*, 587–596. [CrossRef]
14. Kril, V.; Aïqui-Reboul-Paviet, O.; Briant, L.; Amara, A. New Insights into Chikungunya Virus Infection and Pathogenesis. *Annu. Rev. Virol.* **2021**, *8*, 327–347. [CrossRef] [PubMed]
15. Page, M.J.; McKenzie, J.E.; Bossuyt, P.M.; Boutron, I.; Hoffmann, T.C.; Mulrow, C.D.; Shamseer, L.; Tetzlaff, J.M.; Akl, E.A.; Brennan, S.E.; et al. The PRISMA 2020 Statement: An Updated Guideline for Reporting Systematic Reviews. *BMJ* **2021**, *372*, n71. [CrossRef]
16. Wells, G.A.; Shea, B.; O'Connell, D.A.; Peterson, J.; Welch, V.; Losos, M.; Tugwell, P.; The Ottawa Hospital Research Institute. The Newcastle-Ottawa Scale (NOS) for Assessing the Quality of Nonrandomised Studies in Meta-Analyses. 2009. Available online: http://www.ohri.ca/programs/clinical_epidemiology/oxford.asp (accessed on 14 September 2024).
17. Munn, Z.; Barker, T.H.; Moola, S.; Tufanaru, C.; Stern, C.; McArthur, A.; Stephenson, M.; Aromataris, E. Methodological Quality of Case Series Studies: An Introduction to the JBI Critical Appraisal Tool. *JBI Evid. Synth.* **2020**, *18*, 2127–2133. [CrossRef]
18. Moola, S.; Munn, Z.; Tufanaru, C.; Aromataris, E.; Sears, K.; Sfetcu, R.; Currie, M.; Qureshi, R.; Mattis, P.; Lisy, K.; et al. Chapter 7: Systematic Reviews of Etiology and Risk. In *JBI Manual for Evidence Synthesis*; Aromataris, E., Munn, Z., Eds.; JBI: Adelaide, Australia, 2020. Available online: https://synthesismanual.jbi.global (accessed on 14 September 2024).
19. Sterne, J.A.C.; Savović, J.; Page, M.J.; Elbers, R.G.; Blencowe, N.S.; Boutron, I.; Cates, C.J.; Cheng, H.-Y.; Corbett, M.S.; Eldridge, S.M.; et al. RoB 2: A Revised Tool for Assessing Risk of Bias in Randomised Trials. *BMJ* **2019**, *366*, l4898. [CrossRef] [PubMed]
20. Hayd, R.L.N.; Moreno, M.R.; Naveca, F.; Amdur, R.; Suchowiecki, K.; Watson, H.; Firestein, G.S.; Simon, G.; Chang, A.Y. Persistent Chikungunya Arthritis in Roraima, Brazil. *Clin. Rheumatol.* **2020**, *39*, 2781–2787. [CrossRef] [PubMed]
21. Tritsch, S.R.; Encinales, L.; Pacheco, N.; Cadena, A.; Cure, C.; McMahon, E.; Watson, H.; Ramirez, A.P.; Mendoza, A.R.; Li, G.; et al. Chronic Joint Pain 3 Years After Chikungunya Virus Infection Largely Characterized by Relapsing-Remitting Symptoms. *J. Rheumatol.* **2020**, *47*, 1267–1274. [CrossRef]
22. Hossain, S.; Choudhury, M.R.; Islam, M.A.; Hassan, M.; Yeasmin, S.; Hossain, F.; Zaman, M.M. Post-Chikungunya Arthritis: A Longitudinal Study in a Tertiary Care Hospital in Bangladesh. *Trop. Med. Health* **2022**, *50*, 21. [CrossRef] [PubMed]
23. Pollett, S.; Hsieh, H.C.; Lu, D.; Grance, M.; Richard, S.; Nowak, G.; Lanteri, C.; Tribble, D.; Burgess, T. The Risk and Risk Factors of Chikungunya Virus Infection and Rheumatological Sequelae in a Cohort of U.S. Military Health System Beneficiaries: Implications for the Vaccine Era. *PLoS Negl. Trop. Dis.* **2024**, *18*, e0011810. [CrossRef]
24. Bouquillard, E.; Fianu, A.; Bangil, M.; Charlette, N.; Ribéra, A.; Michault, A.; Favier, F.; Simon, F.; Flipo, R.-M. Rheumatic Manifestations Associated with Chikungunya Virus Infection: A Study of 307 Patients with 32-Month Follow-Up (RHUMATOCHIK Study). *Jt. Bone Spine* **2018**, *85*, 207–210. [CrossRef] [PubMed]
25. Manimunda, S.P.; Vijayachari, P.; Uppoor, R.; Sugunan, A.P.; Singh, S.S.; Rai, S.K.; Sudeep, A.B.; Muruganandam, N.; Chaitanya, I.K.; Guruprasad, D.R. Clinical Progression of Chikungunya Fever During Acute and Chronic Arthritic Stages and the Changes in Joint Morphology as Revealed by Imaging. *Trans. R. Soc. Trop. Med. Hyg.* **2010**, *104*, 392–399. [CrossRef] [PubMed]
26. Paul, B.J.; Pannarkady, G.; Moni, S.P.; Thachil, E.J. Clinical Profile and Long-Term Sequelae of Chikungunya Fever. *Indian J. Rheumatol.* **2011**, *6*, 12–19. [CrossRef]
27. Mathew, A.J.; Goyal, V.; George, E.; Thekkemuriyil, D.V.; Jayakumar, B.; Chopra, A.; Trivandrum COPCORD Study Group. Rheumatic-Musculoskeletal Pain and Disorders in a Naïve Group of Individuals 15 Months Following a Chikungunya Viral Epidemic in South India: A Population-Based Observational Study. *Int. J. Clin. Pract.* **2011**, *65*, 1306–1312. [CrossRef] [PubMed]
28. Segura-Charry, J.S.; Parada-Martinez, M.A.; Segura-Puello, H.R.; Muñoz-Forero, D.M.; Nieto-Mosquera, D.L.; Villamil-Ballesteros, A.C.; Cortés-Muñoz, A.J. Musculoskeletal Disorders Due to Chikungunya Virus: A Real Experience in a Rheumatology Department in Neiva, Huila. *Reumatol. Clin.* **2021**, *17*, 456–460. [CrossRef] [PubMed]
29. Rodriguez-Morales, A.J.; Gil-Restrepo, A.F.; Ramírez-Jaramillo, V.; Montoya-Arias, C.P.; Acevedo-Mendoza, W.F.; Bedoya-Arias, J.E.; Chica-Quintero, L.A.; Murillo-García, D.R.; García-Robledo, J.E.; Castrillón-Spitia, J.D.; et al. Post-Chikungunya Chronic Inflammatory Rheumatism: Results from a Retrospective Follow-Up Study of 283 Adult and Child Cases in La Virginia, Risaralda, Colombia. *F1000Res.* **2016**, *5*, 360. [CrossRef]

30. Guillot, X.; Ribera, A.; Gasque, P. Chikungunya-Induced Arthritis in Reunion Island: A Long-Term Observational Follow-Up Study Showing Frequently Persistent Joint Symptoms, Some Cases of Persistent Chikungunya Immunoglobulin M Positivity, and no Anticyclic Citrullinated Peptide Seroconversion After 13 Years. *J. Infect. Dis.* **2020**, *222*, 1740–1744. [CrossRef] [PubMed]
31. Miner, J.J.; Aw-Yeang, H.X.; Fox, J.M.; Taffner, S.; Malkova, O.N.; Oh, S.T.; Kim, A.H.J.; Diamond, M.S.; Lenschow, D.J.; Yokoyama, W.M. Chikungunya Viral Arthritis in the United States: A Mimic of Seronegative Rheumatoid Arthritis. *Arthritis Rheumatol.* **2015**, *67*, 1214–1220. [CrossRef] [PubMed]
32. Bouquillard, E.; Combe, B. A Report of 21 Cases of Rheumatoid Arthritis Following Chikungunya Fever: A Mean Follow-Up of Two Years. *Joint Bone Spine* **2009**, *76*, 654–657. [CrossRef] [PubMed]
33. Javelle, E.; Ribera, A.; Degasne, I.; Gaüzère, B.A.; Marimoutou, C.; Simon, F. Specific Management of Post-Chikungunya Rheumatic Disorders: A Retrospective Study of 159 Cases in Reunion Island from 2006–2012. *PLoS Negl. Trop. Dis.* **2015**, *9*, e0003603. [CrossRef]
34. Amaral, J.K.; Bingham, C.O., 3rd; Schoen, R.T. Successful Methotrexate Treatment of Chronic Chikungunya Arthritis. *J. Clin. Rheumatol.* **2020**, *26*, 119–124. [CrossRef]
35. Ravindran, V.; Alias, G. Efficacy of Combination DMARD Therapy vs. Hydroxychloroquine Monotherapy in Chronic Persistent Chikungunya Arthritis: A 24-Week Randomized Controlled Open Label Study. *Clin. Rheumatol.* **2017**, *36*, 1335–1340. [CrossRef]
36. Rodríguez-Morales, A.J.; Cardona-Ospina, J.A.; Urbano-Garzón, S.F.; Hurtado-Zapata, S. Prevalence of Post-Chikungunya Infection Chronic Inflammatory Arthritis: A Systematic Review and Meta-Analysis. *Arthritis Care Res.* **2016**, *68*, 1849–1858. [CrossRef]
37. Edington, F.; Varjão, D.; Melo, P. Incidence of Articular Pain and Arthritis After Chikungunya Fever in the Americas: A Systematic Review of the Literature and Meta-Analysis. *Jt. Bone Spine* **2018**, *85*, 669–678. [CrossRef] [PubMed]
38. Rama, K.; de Roo, A.M.; Louwsma, T.; Hofstra, H.S.; Amaral, G.S.G.D.; Vondeling, G.T.; Postma, M.J.; Freriks, R.D. Clinical Outcomes of Chikungunya: A Systematic Literature Review and Meta-Analysis. *PLoS Negl. Trop. Dis.* **2024**, *18*, e0012254. [CrossRef] [PubMed]
39. Paixão, E.S.; Rodrigues, L.C.; Costa, M.D.C.N.; Itaparica, M.; Barreto, F.; Gérardin, P.; Teixeira, M.G. Chikungunya Chronic Disease: A Systematic Review and Meta-Analysis. *Trans. R. Soc. Trop. Med. Hyg.* **2018**, *112*, 301–316. [CrossRef] [PubMed]
40. Rodrigo, C.; Herath, T.; Wickramarachchi, U.; Fernando, D.; Rajapakse, S. Treatment of Chikungunya-Associated Joint Pain: A Systematic Review of Controlled Clinical Trials. *Trans. R. Soc. Trop. Med. Hyg.* **2022**, *116*, 889–899. [CrossRef] [PubMed]

Tropical Medicine and Infectious Disease

MDPI

Article

Estimation and Characterization of Dengue Serotypes in Patients Presenting with Dengue Fever at Makkah Hospitals

Sami Melebari [1], Abdul Hafiz [2,*], Hatim A. Natto [3], Mohamed Osman Elamin [4], Naif A. Jalal [2], Ashwaq Hakim [1], Safiah Rushan [5], Othman Fallatah [5], Kamal Alzabeedi [6], Feras Malibari [7], Hutaf Mashat [1], Aisha Alsaadi [1], Amani Alhakam [1], Anoud Hadidi [1], Ghazi Saad Alkhaldi [8], Ahmed Alkhyami [5], Ali Alqarni [5], Abdulaziz Alzahrani [5], Mohammed Alghamdi [5], Abdullah Siddiqi [9], Abdullah Alasmari [10], Rowaida Bakri [2], Saleh Alqahtani [10], Juman M. Al-Bajaly [10] and Asim Khogeer [10,11]

1 Department of Molecular Biology, The Regional Laboratory, Ministry of Health, Makkah 21955, Saudi Arabia; samelibari@yahoo.com (S.M.); athakim@moh.gov.sa (A.H.); hmmashat@moh.gov.sa (H.M.); aialsaadi@moh.gov.sa (A.A.); aalhakam@moh.gov.sa (A.A.); ahadidi@moh.gov.sa (A.H.)

2 Department of Microbiology and Parasitology, Faculty of Medicine, Umm Al-Qura University, Makkah 21955, Saudi Arabia; najalal@uqu.edu.sa (N.A.J.); rabakari@uqu.edu.sa (R.B.)

3 Department of Epidemiology and Biostatistics, Faculty of Public Health & Informatics, Umm Al-Qura University, Makkah 21955, Saudi Arabia; hanatto@uqu.edu.sa

4 Department of Environmental and Occupational Health, Faculty of Public Health and Informatics, Umm Al-Qura University, Makkah 21955, Saudi Arabia; mobushara@uqu.edu.sa

5 Department of Serology, The Regional Laboratory, Ministry of Health, Makkah 21955, Saudi Arabia; srushan@moh.gov.sa (S.R.); ofallatah@moh.gov.sa (O.F.); aalkhyami@moh.gov.sa (A.A.); aaalgarni@moh.gov.sa (A.A.); aalzahrani737@moh.gov.sa (A.A.); moabal-ghamdi@moh.gov.sa (M.A.)

6 Departments of Medical Research, Clinical Biochemistry, The Regional Laboratory, Ministry of Health, Makkah 21955, Saudi Arabia; kalzabeedi@moh.gov.sa

7 Epidemiology and Infection Control, Saudi German Hospital, Makkah 21955, Saudi Arabia; epi.feras@gmail.com

8 Department of Immunology, The Regional Laboratory, Ministry of Health, Makkah 21955, Saudi Arabia; gsalkhaldi@moh.gov.sa

9 Department of Clinical Laboratory, Makkah Park Clinics, Makkah 21955, Saudi Arabia; a.siddiqi@makkahparkclinics.sa

10 Department of Research, PMO, Ministry Branch in Makkah Region, Ministry of Health (MOH), Makkah 21955, Saudi Arabia; aal-asmri@moh.gov.sa (A.A.); sal-qahtani@moh.gov.sa (S.A.); jalbajaly@moh.gov.sa (J.M.A.-B.); akhogeer@moh.gov.sa (A.K.)

11 Medical Genetics Unit, Maternity & Children Hospital, Makkah Healthcare Cluster, Ministry of Health (MOH), Makkah 21955, Saudi Arabia

* Correspondence: aaahafiz@uqu.edu.sa

Abstract: Dengue fever is caused by four common serotypes of the dengue virus (DENV-1, DENV-2, DENV-3, and DENV-4). Patients infected with one serotype may develop lifelong serotype-specific protective immunity. However, they remain susceptible to reinfection with the other serotypes, often increasing the risk of severe forms of dengue. This cross-sectional study investigates the prevalence of the four dengue serotypes in patients who presented with dengue fever at Makkah hospitals between April 2023 and May 2024. Data were collected from the medical records of the Regional Laboratory in Makkah, Saudi Arabia. The 238 positive dengue samples included 185 samples (77.73%) from male patients. The average age of the patients was 37.65 years (SD = 15.05). Dengue type 2 was the most common serotype, followed by type 1, type 3, and type 4. Most of the dengue patients were Saudi nationals, followed by Egyptians. There were 11 dengue-positive samples that were not diagnosed with any of the four dengue serotypes. Since Makkah receives numerous international travelers, these samples might contain novel dengue serotypes circulating in different parts of the world. This study underscores the need for the continuous monitoring of dengue serotypes to predict potential outbreaks and mitigate the risk of severe dengue in susceptible populations.

https://doi.org/10.3390/tropicalmed10010027

Keywords: dengue; Ades; DENV; travel

1. Introduction

Dengue is a mosquito-borne viral disease caused by the dengue virus (DENV) that has enormous public health significance. DENVs belong to the Flaviviridae family of single-stranded RNA viruses that have a positive genetic strand. Almost half of the world's population lives in areas at risk of dengue infection. An estimated 100–400 million people are infected with the dengue virus annually [1]. However, only a few of these infections develop into clinical cases. In 2023, there were an estimated 6.5 million cases of dengue, and it caused 6800 deaths globally [2]. In the WHO East Mediterranean Region, dengue is endemic in Afghanistan, Djibouti, Egypt, Oman, Pakistan, Saudi Arabia, Somalia, Sudan, and Yemen. Two vector species are involved in DENV transmission in this region: *Ae. aegypti*, which is the primary vector, and *Ae. albopictus*, which is considered to be the secondary vector [3].

Dengue is more common in tropical and subtropical regions. However, due to environmental changes and increased global travel and transportation, mosquito vectors have established themselves in newer locations, and thus has the dengue virus [4]. Most DENV infections may be subclinical or asymptomatic and thus remain undiagnosed. In the majority of dengue cases, the illness first causes a moderate fever, but after three to fifteen days, the infected person may experience various symptoms, including a very high temperature [5,6]. However, a small percentage of dengue infections may turn into severe, life-threatening conditions. The progression of dengue disease from non-severe to severe forms, such as Dengue Hemorrhagic Fever (DHF) or Dengue Shock Syndrome (DSS), is influenced by multiple factors. Understanding these factors is crucial for predicting and managing severe dengue cases [7–9]. Key factors include the infecting viral serotype, host immune history and status, environmental conditions, and the timing of medical intervention or access to healthcare.

Dengue virus infections elicit serotype-specific host immune responses [10,11]. There are four distinct serotypes of the dengue virus, known as DENV-1, DENV-2, DENV-3, and DENV-4, and they are detected quite frequently [12]. However, a rare fifth serotype has also been reported [13]. The distinct dengue virus serotypes share over 65% of their genomic identity and are genetically related [14–16], meaning they differ in their antigenic properties but are closely related enough to cause similar clinical symptoms. While infection with any one serotype typically provides long-lasting immunity against that specific serotype, it may not help elicit a protective immune response against the other serotypes. In fact, subsequent infection with a different serotype can lead to more severe forms of the disease [17]. DENV-2 is frequently linked to more serious outcomes, especially in secondary infections. Several factors contribute to the severity of DENV-2, including antibody-dependent enhancement of the infection, making DENV-2 one of the most virulent serotypes from a public health perspective [17–19].

In addition, DENV-5, a new serotype of the dengue virus, was reported in 2013 [20,21]. However, this new serotype has not yet been approved by the International Committee on Taxonomy of Viruses (ICTV). The discovery of DENV-5 highlights the complexity of dengue virus transmission and evolution. While this serotype has not yet caused widespread human outbreaks, its presence underscores the need for continued surveillance and research to better understand its potential impact on public health [21].

Dengue is considered an endemic disease in certain regions of Saudi Arabia, such as the western and southwestern coastal areas, including the cities of Jeddah, Makkah, and

Medina. These regions have favorable climates for the mosquito *Aedes aegypti*, which is the primary vector for the dengue virus in the area [22–25]. The Saudi Arabian government, through the Ministry of Health (MOH), has implemented control measures to combat dengue, including mosquito control programs, public health campaigns, and surveillance systems [26]. Despite these efforts, dengue outbreaks still occur in rainy seasons as well as sporadically [27]. In addition, the city of Makkah receives millions of visitors from different parts of the world, including areas that are dengue endemic zones, to perform prayers and undertake *Umrah* and *Hajj*. It is important to monitor the dengue serotypes circulating in this city to help dengue control efforts in Makkah as well as in Saudi Arabia in general [28].

The purpose of this study is to examine reported cases of dengue in Makkah; determine the age, gender, and nationality distribution of these dengue cases; and identify the dengue serotypes present in the city.

2. Materials and Methods

2.1. Study Site and Population

Makkah is a city of religious importance in Islam located in Saudi Arabia. *Al-Masjid Al-Haram*, the most important *Masjid* in Islam, is situated in Makkah. Millions of Muslims travel to Makkah from different parts of the world every year. It is Saudi Arabia's third most populous metropolis. In 2023, Makkah's population was 2 million. The population fluctuates significantly during the *Hijri* months of *Ramadan* and the annual *Hajj* pilgrimage as millions of Muslims from around the world travel to Makkah. During the month of *Ramadan* and the *Hajj* pilgrimage, the population of this city can swell, increasing by a few million additional people, reflecting the massive influx of pilgrims [29]. Makkah's climate is hot in the summer, often being more than 40 °C during the day and dipping to 30 °C at night. Nonetheless, it is mild during the winter, with daytime highs of 30 °C and nighttime lows of 18 °C. Makkah often receives a few inches of rain between November and January which may cause fluctuations in the dengue-vector population [28,30,31].

2.2. Study Design

This is a cross-sectional data analysis study. We enrolled laboratory-confirmed dengue patients from Makkah hospitals between April 2023 and May 2024. Patients with negative dengue diagnoses in the laboratory were excluded. The dengue case definition used in this study was in accordance with the Ministry of Health, Saudi Arabia [32,33]. This study's participants were Makkah city residents, citizens, and travelers/visitors who had been diagnosed with dengue at Makkah hospitals. Demographic details, including age, gender, and nationality, were collected from the healthcare-providing hospitals.

2.3. Criteria for Suspected and Confirmed Dengue Cases

A suspected dengue case was defined as a person with acute febrile illness or a history of acute febrile illness for the past 2–7 days, plus two or more of the additional dengue symptoms as determined by a physician. These additional symptoms include headache, arthralgia, retro-orbital pain, myalgia, rash, leucopenia, and hemorrhagic manifestations [34]. A confirmed dengue case was defined as a person whose sample was identified as positive via quantitative reverse transcription polymerase chain reaction (RT-qPCR) during dengue diagnosis.

2.4. Collecting Samples

Samples from all suspected dengue cases were collected from Makkah hospitals and were forwarded to the regional laboratory in Makkah to test for anti-dengue immunoglobulins (IgMs) using an enzyme-linked immunoassay (ELISA) and the dengue virus RNA via polymerase chain reaction (RT-PCR), as described in the protocol [34]. The results were recorded on the HESN plus webpage. The Saudi Arabian Ministry of Health (MOH) requires all its laboratories to record laboratory results on this webpage. The HESN is part of MOH's Epidemiological Surveillance Program [35]. For further molecular studies, the materials were maintained at −80 °C in constant freezing conditions.

2.5. Extraction of Ribonucleic Acid (RNA)

RNA was extracted from 300 μL of a serum specimen utilizing a MagNA Pure 96 Instrument (Roche Molecular Systems, Inc., Mannheim, Germany) according to the instructions provided by the manufacturer.

2.6. Quantitative Reverse Transcription Polymerase Chain Reaction (RT-qPCR) and Reverse Transcription Polymerase Chain Reaction (RT-PCR)

The RT-qPCR tests were performed using a LightMix Modular Dengue Virus kit (Roche Diagnostics (Schweiz) AG), as per the instructions given by the manufacturer. Precisely 10 μL of the reaction mixture was added to 10 μL of the purified RNA. The PCR reaction per well included 4.0 μL of Roche master; 0.1 μL of the RT enzyme; 0.5 μL of the reagent mix, including primers and probes; and 5.4 μL of PCR-grade water. The reverse transcription phase was completed using the following parameters: a 55 °C RT step for 5 min, and then 95 °C denaturation for 5 min, followed by 45 cycles of 5 s at 95 °C, 15 s at 60 °C, and 15 s at 72 °C in quantification mode. Finally, the reaction was cooled at 40 °C for 30 s. All procedures were performed in a LightCycler 480 instrument, and results were analyzed using the LightCycler software 480 (Roche Molecular Systems, Inc., Germany). RT-PCR was used for serotyping. The procedure was similar to RT-qPCR except that a Realstar® Dengue Type RT-PCR Kit 1.0 from Altona Diagnostics was used, as per the instructions supplied with the kit. The kit does not use any housekeeping gene probe for internal control; instead, it uses a heterologous amplification system as an internal control to identify possible RT-PCR inhibition and confirm the integrity of the reagents of the kit. Since it uses a "heterologous amplification system" instead of a housekeeping gene as an internal control, this kit cannot determine the integrity of RNA obtained from a patient. It can only determine the integrity of the reagents of the kit and the inhibition of the RT-PCR reaction.

2.7. Enzyme-Linked Immunosorbent Assay (ELISA)

The ELISA method was utilized to qualitatively detect the NS1 antigen (Platelia™ Dengue NS1 Ag, Bio-RAD, Marnes-la-Coquette, France) and IgG and IgM human antibodies against DENV (SERION ELISA classic, Dengue Virus IgG/IgM). All the internal controls and samples given in each kit were treated according to the manufacturer's instructions, using a completely automated ELISA system. (Human Diagnostics, Wiesbaden, Germany).

2.8. Statistical Analysis

Data were input into Microsoft Excel spreadsheets. The data inputs were double-checked to eliminate any data entry errors. All data analysis and curve plotting for data display were performed using Microsoft Excel.

3. Results

A total of 238 positive dengue samples were studied from April 2023 to May 2024. Of these samples, 77.73% (n = 185) and 22.27% (n = 53) were from male and female patients, respectively. The average age of the patients was 37.65 years (standard deviation = 15.05). The average Ct value for RT-qPCR was 27.33 (standard deviation = 4.35). Serological tests revealed that 81.51% of the analyzed samples were positive for the NS1 antigen ELISA (n = 194), 78.57% were positive for the IgM antibody ELISA (n = 187), and 44.53% were positive for the IgG antibody ELISA (n = 106) (Table 1). There were differences in the serological findings and RT-qPCR Ct values between male and female patients (Table 1). Male patients were greater in number than female patients in all but three hospitals (Table A1). SUHAIL hospital, which caters to patients coming for *Hajj* and *Umrah* near *Al-Masjid Al-Haram*, reported the highest number of male and female patients (Table A1).

Table 1. The general and laboratory characteristics of the study samples.

	All Samples (n = 238)	Non 1,2,3,4 Serotype (n = 11)	Samples from Male Patients (n = 185)	Samples from Female Patients (n = 53)
Average age (St Dev)	37.65 (15.05)	33.9 (14.63)	36.83 (13.89)	40.49 (18.12)
Gender (male patients)	77.73%	72.72%	100%	0%
NS1 reactive	81.51%	81.81%	83.78%	73.58%
IgM reactive	78.57%	72.72%	80.54%	71.69%
IgG reactive	44.53%	54.54%	43.78%	47.16%
Average Ct (St Dev)	27.33 (4.35)	26.21 (8.00)	26.85 (3.99)	28.99 (5.16)

The study period comprised sixty weeks (fourteen months). However, dengue cases were observed only for a total of seventeen weeks. The DENV2 serotype was detected throughout these seventeen weeks, while DENV1 was found in weeks 14, 18, 25, 26, 27, and 28 of 2023 and weeks 18 and 21 of 2024. Most of the non 1,2,3,4 serotype samples were diagnosed in weeks 14 and 18 of 2023 (Figure 1).

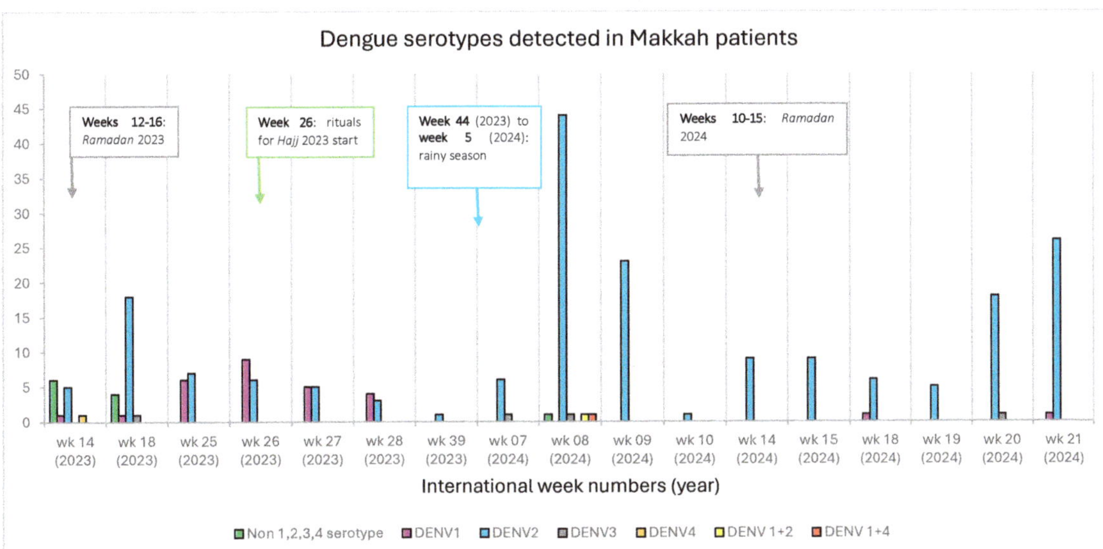

Figure 1. Dengue serotypes detected in different weeks in 2023 and 2024. The different colored bars show the number of various dengue serotypes detected according to international weeks in 2023 and 2024. The weeks pertaining to the month of *Ramadan* in 2023 (22 March–20 April), the month of *Ramadan* in 2024 (10 March–09 April), the start date of *Hajj* rituals (26 June 2023), and the rainy season in Makkah (November–January) are marked with different colored arrows.

Patients of several nationalities were found to be dengue-positive (Table 2). Saudi patients accounted for 40.34% of the total (n = 96) followed by 18.07% (n = 43) patients from Egypt, 9.24% (n = 22) from Pakistan, and 5.88% (n = 14) of unknown nationalities. Bangladesh and India each accounted for 5.04% (n = 12) of confirmed cases. Yemen accounted for 4.62% (n = 11) of the total dengue cases. Myanmar and Sudan accounted for 2.94% (n = 7) of the patients. Afghanistan, Algeria, and Iraq contributed to 1.26% (n = 3) of cases. Syria accounted for 0.84% of cases (n = 2) while Mali, Nepal, and Tunisia accounted for 0.42% of the cases (n = 1).

Table 2. Dengue serotypes and nationalities of the patients. Dengue serotype 2 was the most common, followed by type 1. There were 11 samples that did not react to the detection kits for types 1, 2, 3, or 4 (non 1, 2, 3, and 4 type). Two cases of mixed serotype infections were also detected.

Nationality	Dengue Type							Total	% of Total
	Type 1	Type 2	Type 3	Type 4	Non 1,2,3,4	Type 1 + 2	Type 1 + 4		
Saudi Arabia	13	75	2	1	4	1	-	96	40.34
Egypt	2	38	1		2	-	-	43	18.07
Pakistan	-	18	1		3	-	-	22	9.24
Unknown	1	12	-	-	-	-	1	14	5.88
Bangladesh	-	12	-	-	-	-	-	12	5.04
India	4	8	-	-	-	-	-	12	5.04
Yemen	2	8	-	-	1	-		11	4.62
Myanmar	-	7	-	-	-	-	-	7	2.94
Sudan	2	4	-	-	1	-	-	7	2.94
Afghanistan	1	2	-	-	-	-	-	3	1.26
Algeria	2	1	-	-	-	-	-	3	1.26
Iraq	2	1	-	-	-	-	-	3	1.26
Syria	-	2	-	-	-	-	-	2	0.84
Mali	-	1	-	-	-	-	-	1	0.42
Nepal	-	1	-	-	-	-	-	1	0.42
Tunisia	-	1	-	-	-	-	-	1	0.42
Total	29	191	4	1	11	1	1	238	100.00

An age distribution analysis was conducted to determine the distribution of dengue infection by age (Table 3). The 21–30-year-old and 31–40-year-old age groups each accounted for 26.89% of the total dengue cases (n = 64, each). The 41–50 age group accounted for 15.97% of cases (n = 38), followed by the 51–60 age group, which accounted for 12.18% (n = 29).

Table 3. Dengue cases arranged by age group. Mixed infections were only observed in the 41–50 age group. The non 1, 2, 3, 4 serotype had a broad distribution in all age groups, except for those 11–20 years of age and 70+ years old.

Age Groups	Dengue Type							Total	% of Total
	Type 1	Type 2	Type 3	Type 4	Non 1,2,3,4	Type 1 + 2	Type 1 + 4		
0–10 years	-	4	-	-	1	-	-	5	2.10
11–20 years	4	12	1	-	-	-	-	17	7.14
21–30 years	6	52	2	-	4	-	-	64	26.89
31–40 years	3	59	-	1	1	-	-	64	26.89
41–50 years	6	27	-		3	1	1	38	15.97
51–60 years	6	21	1	-	1	-	-	29	12.18
61–70 years	1	12	-	-	1	-	-	14	5.88
70+ years	2	5	-	-	-	-	-	7	2.94
Total	28	192	4	1	11	1	1	238	100.00

All four main dengue serotypes reported in Saudi Arabia were also detected in our patients. Dengue type 2 was detected in 80.25% of patients (n = 191), followed by serotype 1 in 12.18% (n = 29), serotype 3 in 1.68% (n = 4), and serotype 4 in 0.42% (n = 1) of our study patients. However, about 4.62% (n = 11) of the patients were infected with a dengue serotype that could not be identified in our assays. In these 11 samples, 81.81% were reactive to NS1 antigen, 72.72% were reactive to IgM, and 54.54% were reactive to IgG antibodies in serological dengue diagnostic tests. The reactivity in serological tests for NS1 and IgM, the gender distribution, the average ages, and the average Ct values for these 11 samples were similar to those of the total study samples. However, reactivity to IgG was higher in these 11 samples compared to the total samples (54.54% vs. 44.53%) (Table 1).

4. Discussion

The city of Makkah in the Kingdom of Saudi Arabia receives millions of local and international travelers every year. Makkah has a population of 2 million. It received almost 1.8 million *Hajj* pilgrims in 2024. More than 10 million *Umrah* performers visited *Al-Masjid Al-Haram* in the *Hijri* month of *Ramadan* in 2022 [29]. In addition, millions of foreigners live in the Kingdom as residents. Infectious diseases come with the local and international travelers to Makkah. These travelers come from almost every part of the world. The city of Makkah has been receiving international travelers since ancient times, impacting almost all aspects of human life including public health. In the past, the influx of foreign religious travelers was limited, as international travel was not as fast and convenient as it is these days. In modern times, the number of *Umrah* and *Hajj* travelers has considerably increased.

The bulk of travelers to Makkah come in the *Hijri* months of *Ramadan* and *Dhul-Hijjah* (the month of *Hajj*). These visitors may come to Makkah a few weeks before these months, and some stay a few weeks after the end of this period. It is quite interesting to note that the non-1, -2, -3, or -4 serotypes and DENV1 were diagnosed in and around the months of *Ramadan* and *Dhul Hijjah*. No dengue cases were diagnosed during the annual rainy season from November to January. However, the highest number of dengue-positive samples in Makkah were diagnosed two weeks after the end of the rainy season, implicating rain in the transmission of this mosquito-borne disease. Vector-born disease transmission patterns are influenced by several environmental factors, including rain, changes in land use, human movements, and so on [36,37].

Our study suggests that most of the dengue patients were Saudi nationals who could have been Makkah residents or had come to Makkah from different parts of the country. Dengue is endemic in Saudi Arabia [24]. The infections were more common in adult males between 21 and 30 and 31 and 40 years old.

More male than female patients were diagnosed with dengue in Makkah during the study period. This phenomenon has been reported in several previous studies [36,37]. Moreover, dengue was less prevalent in children and the elderly. Females, children, and the elderly may not be exposed to mosquito bites in the same proportion as adult males who are regularly engaged in fieldwork. In Makkah, foreign men come more frequently than women for *Umrah*, *Hajj*, and work. Cleaners, construction workers, security personnel, and vehicle drivers that transport visitors and goods from other cities to Makkah are also mostly male. Studies characterizing the professions and socio-economic statuses of dengue patients may provide interesting insights into dengue transmission patterns.

A comparison between the two gender groups in our study shows that women had higher Ct values, higher proportions of IgG-reactive samples, and lower proportions of NS1- and IgM-reactive samples than men. This suggests that women might have been diagnosed with dengue infection later as compared to men in our study. There might be differences in the health-seeking behaviors of the two genders. Such gender-based differences in the number of reported dengue cases are consistently observed in multiple culturally and economically different countries [38,39]. It should be noted that only an estimated 1–6% of dengue infections develop into clinical cases [2]. It would be interesting to determine if there are gender-associated determinants of dengue disease manifestation or severity. The gender differences observed in this study warrant further investigation into potential behavioral or biological factors.

Interestingly, 11 of our dengue-positive samples did not react to type-1-, -2-, -3-, or -4-specific RT-PCR assays. The general and laboratory characteristics of these 11 samples were comparable to those of the total study samples, suggesting there are no other anomalies in the laboratory findings for these samples. The average Ct value of the RT-qPCR was also comparable with that of the total samples. However, the possibility of template degradation or the presence of PCR inhibitors in the samples during serotyping RT-PCR remains. Since Makkah receives millions of global visitors, the presence of novel or rare dengue serotypes cannot be ruled out either. Further studies with molecular and viral genome-sequencing approaches are needed to determine the presence of novel dengue serotypes.

The study had several limitations; therefore, the results should be interpreted with caution. Firstly, we recruited only suspected dengue patients presenting at various hospitals in Makkah. Therefore, this study does not reflect on the total number of dengue infections in Makkah. Secondly, not all dengue cases diagnosed among foreigners are traveler's infections. Several foreigners live in Saudi Arabia for work and business as residents. Finally, people may have altered health-seeking behavior when they travel as compared to when they are at the comfort of their homes. Similarly, there may be differences in health-seeking behavior among people of different genders, age groups, social as well as economic groups.

5. Conclusions

Dengue is endemic in Saudi Arabia. We observed 238 dengue cases during the study period. Most of the dengue patients in our study were Saudi nationals. In addition to the prompt diagnosis and treatment of dengue cases, continuous case surveillance and vector control efforts are important to contain the disease in Makkah. Dengue serotype 2 was the most prevalent serotype in Makkah during the study period. Dengue was more frequently diagnosed in males than females. It would be quite interesting to determine the underlying causes for this observed gender-based difference. We could not determine the dengue serotypes in the samples collected from 11 patients. Further research is needed to confirm the presence of uncommon or rare dengue serotypes in Makkah.

Author Contributions: Conceptualization, A.H. (Abdul Hafiz) and S.M.; methodology, A.K., H.M., A.A. (Ahmed Alkhyami) and R.B.; software, A.A. (Abdulaziz Alzahrani), A.A. (Amani Alhakam), A.S., S.A. and F.M.; validation, M.O.E., R.B., A.S. and H.M.; formal analysis, A.H. (Abdul Hafiz), A.K. and M.O.E.; investigation, S.M., A.H. (Anoud Hadidi), A.A. (Ali Alqarni) and H.A.N.; resources, F.M., A.A. (Aisha Alsaadi), A.A. (Abdullah Alasmarii) and A.H. (Ashwaq Hakim); data curation, A.A. (Ahmed Alkhyami), A.S., J.M.A.-B., O.F. and G.S.A.; writing—original draft preparation, A.H. (Abdul Hafiz) and S.M.; writing—review and editing, A.K., H.A.N., R.B. and M.O.E.; visualization, N.A.J., S.R., M.A., S.A. and A.K.; supervision, S.M., K.A. and A.H. (Abdul Hafiz); project administration, S.M. and A.K. All authors have read and agreed to the published version of the manuscript.

Funding: This research work was funded by Umm Al-Qura University, Saudi Arabia under grant number 25UQU4350021GSSR01.

Institutional Review Board Statement: This study was approved by the Research Ethics Committee of the Ministry of Health of Saudi Arabia (ethical approval reference no. H-02-K-076-1024-1196, issued in 2024). Confidentiality was maintained throughout the study.

Informed Consent Statement: Not applicable.

Data Availability Statement: Data can be obtained from the corresponding author after approval from the Ministry of Health, Saudi Arabia.

Acknowledgments: The authors extend their appreciation to Umm Al-Qura University, Saudi Arabia for funding this research work through grant number: 25UQU4350021GSSR01.

Conflicts of Interest: The authors declare no conflicts of interest.

Appendix A

Table A1. Dengue cases arranged according to the referring hospital. The number of male and female cases is listed by the name of the referring hospital in Makkah.

Hospital Name	Number of Males	Number of Females
ALAHLI	11	2
ALABEER	1	1
ALBADR	1	-
ALBEYAT MEDICAL	11	-
ALHUDA	3	-
ALRAFIE	1	-
ALSHEFA	1	1
BASHARAHEEL	4	1
HERA	8	8
KING ABDULAZIZ	8	2
KING FISAL	17	8
KHULAIS	2	2
MAKKAH MEDICAL	21	4
MATERNITY&CHILDREN	1	2
ALNOOR	26	3
SAUDI HOSPITAL	5	-
SECURITY FORCES	8	5
SUHAIL	56	10
KING ABDULAZIZ MEDICAL CENTRE	-	3
SAUDI GERMAN	-	1
Total	**185**	**53**

References

1. *Fact Sheet: Dengue and Severe Dengue*; The Worlds Health Organization: Geneva, Switzerland, 2024. Available online: https://www.who.int/news-room/fact-sheets/detail/dengue-and-severe-dengue (accessed on 1 November 2024).
2. Haider, N.; Hasan, M.N.; Onyango, J.; Asaduzzaman, M. Global landmark: 2023 marks the worst year for dengue cases with millions infected and thousands of deaths reported. *IJID Reg.* **2024**, *13*, 100459. [CrossRef]
3. *Dengue Global Situation*; The Worlds Health Organization: Geneva, Switzerland, 2023. Available online: https://www.who.int/emergencies/disease-outbreak-news/item/2023-DON498 (accessed on 1 November 2024).
4. World Health Organization. *Dengue, Countries or Areas at Risk, 2013*; World Health Organization: Geneva, Switzerland, 2014.
5. Anderson, J.R.; Rico-Hesse, R. Aedes aegypti vectorial capacity is determined by the infecting genotype of dengue virus. *Am. J. Trop. Med. Hyg.* **2006**, *75*, 886. [CrossRef]
6. Basurko, C.; Matheus, S.; Hildéral, H.; Everhard, S.; Restrepo, M.; Cuadro-Alvarez, E.; Lambert, V.; Boukhari, R.; Duvernois, J.-P.; Favre, A.; et al. Estimating the risk of vertical transmission of dengue: A prospective study. *Am. J. Trop. Med. Hyg.* **2018**, *98*, 1826. [CrossRef] [PubMed]
7. Santana, L.M.R.; Baquero, O.S.; Maeda, A.Y.; Nogueira, J.S.; Chiaravalloti, F. Spatio-temporal dynamics of dengue-related deaths and associated factors. *Rev. Do Inst. Med. Trop. São Paulo* **2022**, *64*, e30. [CrossRef] [PubMed]
8. Ratnam, I.; Leder, K.; Black, J.; Torresi, J. Dengue fever and international travel. *J. Travel Med.* **2013**, *20*, 384–393. [CrossRef]
9. Rigau-Pérez, J.G.; Clark, G.G.; Gubler, D.J.; Reiter, P.; Sanders, E.J.; Vorndam, A.V. Dengue and dengue haemorrhagic fever. *Lancet* **1998**, *352*, 971–977. [CrossRef]
10. Sabin, A.B. Research on dengue during World War II. *Am. J. Trop. Med. Hyg.* **1952**, *1*, 30–50. [CrossRef] [PubMed]

11. Imrie, A.; Meeks, J.; Gurary, A.; Sukhbaatar, M.; Truong, T.T.; Cropp, C.B.; Effler, P. Antibody to dengue 1 detected more than 60 years after infection. *Viral Immunol.* **2007**, *20*, 672–675. [CrossRef]
12. Hassan, M.; Hassan, A.; Farooq, M.; Afzal, S.; Khan, M.A.; Amin, I.; Shahid, M.; Idrees, M.; Shahid, A.A. Dengue vaccines: Ongoing challenges and current status in the advancement of different candidates. Critical Reviews™ in Eukaryotic Gene. *Expression* **2021**, *31*, 7–19.
13. Sabir, M.J.; Al-Saud, N.B.S.; Hassan, S.M. Dengue and human health: A global scenario of its occurrence, diagnosis and therapeutics. *Saudi J. Biol. Sci.* **2021**, *28*, 5074–5080. [CrossRef] [PubMed]
14. Pintado Silva, J.; Fernandez-Sesma, A. Challenges on the development of a dengue vaccine: A comprehensive review of the state of the art. *J. Gen. Virol.* **2023**, *104*, 001831. [CrossRef] [PubMed]
15. Murugesan, A.; Manoharan, M. Dengue virus. In *Emerging and Reemerging Viral Pathogens*; Elsevier: Amsterdam, The Netherlands, 2020; pp. 281–359.
16. Guzman, M.G.; Gubler, D.J.; Izquierdo, A.; Martinez, E.; Halstead, S.B. Dengue infection. *Nat. Rev. Dis. Primers* **2016**, *2*, 1–25. [CrossRef] [PubMed]
17. Harapan, H.; Michie, A.; Sasmono, R.T.; Imrie, A. Dengue: A minireview. *Viruses* **2020**, *12*, 829. [CrossRef] [PubMed]
18. Fried, J.R.; Gibbons, R.V.; Kalayanarooj, S.; Thomas, S.J.; Srikiatkhachorn, A.; Yoon, I.K.; Jarman, R.G.; Green, S.; Rothman, A.L.; Cummings, D.A. Serotype-specific differences in the risk of dengue hemorrhagic fever: An analysis of data collected in Bangkok, Thailand from 1994 to 2006. *PLoS Neglected Trop. Dis.* **2010**, *4*, e617. [CrossRef]
19. Vicente, C.R.; Herbinger, K.-H.; Fröschl, G.; Malta Romano, C.; de Souza Areias Cabidelle, A.; Cerutti Junior, C. Serotype influences on dengue severity: A cross-sectional study on 485 confirmed dengue cases in Vitória, Brazil. *BMC Infect. Dis.* **2016**, *16*, 320. [CrossRef]
20. Normile, D. *Surprising New Dengue Virus Throws a Spanner in Disease Control Efforts*; American Association for the Advancement of Science: Washington, DC, USA, 2013.
21. Mustafa, M.; Rasotgi, V.; Jain, S.; Gupta, V. Discovery of fifth serotype of dengue virus (DENV-5): A new public health dilemma in dengue control. *Med. J. Armed Forces India* **2015**, *71*, 67–70. [CrossRef] [PubMed]
22. Hafiz, A.; Bakri, R.; Alsaad, M. The World Health Organization's declaration of Egypt as malaria free will boost malaria control efforts in the region. *New Microbes New Infect.* **2024**, *62*, 101529. [CrossRef]
23. Murray, N.E.A.; Quam, M.B.; Wilder-Smith, A. Epidemiology of dengue: Past, present and future prospects. *Clin. Epidemiol.* **2013**, *5*, 299–309.
24. Al-Raddadi, R.; Alwafi, O.; Shabouni, O.; Akbar, N.; Alkhalawi, M.; Ibrahim, A.; Hussain, R.; Alzahrani, M.; Al Helal, M.; Assiri, A. Seroprevalence of dengue fever and the associated sociodemographic, clinical, and environmental factors in Makkah, Madinah, Jeddah, and Jizan, Kingdom of Saudi Arabia. *Acta Trop.* **2019**, *189*, 54–64. [CrossRef]
25. Kanan, M.; Naffaa, M.; Alanazi, A.; Nasser, F.; Alsaiari, A.A.; Almehmadi, M.; Assiry, A.; Muzafar, H.; Katam, H.; Arar, A.; et al. Genetic variants associated with dengue hemorrhagic fever. A systematic review and meta-analysis. *J. Infect. Public Health* **2024**, *17*, 579–587. [CrossRef] [PubMed]
26. Dengue Fever Disease: Guidance for Surveillance, Case Diagnosis, and Management. Public Health Authority, The Kingdom of Saudi Arabia. V.1.3 Edition. 2023. Available online: https://www.pha.gov.sa/Style%20Library/Images/PublicHealthPortal/RiskFactorsDiseases/DengueFever/DengueFever.pdf (accessed on 1 November 2024).
27. Yousuf, R.; Salam, M.W.; Akter, S.; Sinha, S.; Haque, M. Dengue Dynamics: A Global Update. *Adv. Hum. Biol.* **2024**, *14*, 5–10. [CrossRef]
28. Melebari, S.; Bakri, R.; Hafiz, A.; Qabbani, F.; Khogeer, A.; Alharthi, I.; Alhazmi, S.; Almalki, Y.; Bulkhi, R.; Gammash, R.; et al. The epidemiology and incidence of dengue in Makkah, Saudi Arabia, during 2017–2019. *Saudi Med. J.* **2021**, *42*, 1173. [CrossRef] [PubMed]
29. Pilgrims Experience Programme, Annual Report 2023. Available online: https://www.vision2030.gov.sa/media/0hwbcwev/pep-annual-report-2023-english.pdf (accessed on 1 November 2024).
30. Khan, S.; Alghafari, Y. Temperature, precipitation and relative humidity fluctuation of Makkah Al Mukarramah, kingdom of Saudi Arabia (1985–2016). *Trans. Mach. Learn. Artif. Intell.* **2018**, *6*, 42.
31. Melebari, S.; Hafiz, A.; Alzabeedi, K.H.; Alzahrani, A.A.; Almalki, Y.; Jadkarim, R.J.; Qabbani, F.; Bakri, R.; Jalal, N.A.; Mashat, H.; et al. Malaria during COVID-19 Travel Restrictions in Makkah, Saudi Arabia. *Trop. Med. Infect. Dis.* **2024**, *9*, 112. [CrossRef] [PubMed]
32. Rigau-Pérez, J.G.; Gubler, D.J.; Vorndam, A.V.; Clark, G.G. Dengue: A literature review and case study of travelers from the United States, 1986–1994. *J. Travel Med.* **1997**, *4*, 65–71. [CrossRef]
33. Gubler, D. The global pandemic of dengue/dengue haemorrhagic fever: Current status and prospects for the future. *Ann. Acad. Med. Singap.* **1998**, *27*, 227–234. [PubMed]
34. de Oliveira Poersch, C.; Pavoni, D.P.; Queiroz, M.H.; de Borba, L.; Goldenberg, S.; dos Santos, C.N.D.; Krieger, M.A. Dengue virus infections: Comparison of methods for diagnosing the acute disease. *J. Clin. Virol.* **2005**, *32*, 272–277. [CrossRef] [PubMed]

35. Almayahi, Z.K.; Alswaidi, F.; Alzahrani, A. Perception of the health surveillance users on the health electronic surveillance network (HESN), Saudi Arabia, 2016. *J. Egypt. Public Health Assoc.* **2021**, *96*, 17. [CrossRef] [PubMed] [PubMed Central]
36. Swei, A.; Couper, L.I.; Coffey, L.L.; Kapan, D.; Bennett, S. Patterns, Drivers, and Challenges of Vector-Borne Disease Emergence. *Vector Borne Zoonotic Dis.* **2020**, *20*, 159–170. [CrossRef] [PubMed] [PubMed Central]
37. Shamshad, H.; Hafiz, A.; Althagafi, I.I.; Saeed, M.; Mirza, A.Z. Characterization of the *Trypanosoma brucei* Pteridine Reductase Active- Site using Computational Docking and Virtual Screening Techniques. *Curr. Comput.-Aided Drug Des.* **2020**, *16*, 583–598. [CrossRef] [PubMed]
38. Anker, M.; Arima, Y. Male-female differences in the number of reported incident dengue fever cases in six Asian countries. *West. Pac. Surveill. Response J.* **2011**, *2*, 17–23. [CrossRef] [PubMed]
39. Shekhar, K.C.; Huat, O.L. Epidemiology of dengue/dengue hemorrhagic fever in Malaysia--a retrospective epidemiological study 1973–1987. Part I: Dengue hemorrhagic fever (DHF). *Asia-Pac. J. Public Health* **1992**, *6*, 15–25. [CrossRef] [PubMed]

Tropical Medicine and Infectious Disease

MDPI

Review

Suppression of Interferon Response and Antiviral Strategies of Bunyaviruses

Yingying He [1,2,†], Min Shen [1,2,†], Xiaohe Wang [1,2], Anqi Yin [1,2], Bingyan Liu [1], Jie Zhu [1,*] and Zhenhua Zhang [1,*]

1 Institute of Clinical Virology, Department of Infectious Diseases, The Second Affiliated Hospital of Anhui Medical University, Hefei 230601, China; hyy0189@163.com (Y.H.); shenmin200202@163.com (M.S.); wxhwxh2001@outlook.com (X.W.); yaq0127@163.com (A.Y.); lby081921@163.com (B.L.)
2 Department of Clinical Medicine, Anhui Medical University, Hefei 230032, China
* Correspondence: jiezhu0731@gmail.com (J.Z.); zzh1974cn@163.com (Z.Z.)
† These authors contributed equally to this work.

Abstract: The order Bunyavirales belongs to the class of Ellioviricetes and is classified into fourteen families. Some species of the order Bunyavirales pose potential threats to human health. The continuously increasing research reveals that various viruses within this order achieve immune evasion in the host through suppressing interferon (IFN) response. As the types and nodes of the interferon response pathway are continually updated or enriched, the IFN suppression mechanisms and target points of different virus species within this order are also constantly enriched and exhibit variations. For instance, Puumala virus (PUUV) and Tula virus (TULV) can inhibit IFN response through their functional NSs inhibiting downstream factor IRF3 activity. Nevertheless, the IFN suppression mechanisms of Dabie bandavirus (DBV) and Guertu virus (GTV) are mostly mediated by viral inclusion bodies (IBs) or filamentous structures (FSs). Currently, there are no effective drugs against several viruses belonging to this order that pose significant threats to society and human health. While the discovery, development, and application of antiviral drugs constitute a lengthy process, our focus on key targets in the IFN response suppression process of the virus leads to potential antiviral strategies, which provide references for both basic research and practical applications.

Keywords: bunyavirus; interferon; NSs; TBK1; STAT; targeted therapy

1. Introduction

The order Bunyavirales belongs to the class of Ellioviricetes. Over 500 different species of bunyaviruses were described and are widely distributed around the world. They circulate in nature through blood-feeding arthropods and susceptible vertebrates with the capability to infect a variety of animals and plants [1], which leads to significant biosecurity concerns and causes severe economic damage. Among them, some important bunyaviruses, such as Crimean–Congo hemorrhagic fever virus (CCHFV) and Dabie bandavirus (DBV), are primarily transmitted through tick biting, while La Crosse virus (LACV) is mainly transmitted by the Aedes triseriatus mosquito, etc.

According to the International Committee on Taxonomy of Viruses (ICTV), the order Bunyaviridaes currently is divided into fourteen families: Arenaviridae, Cruliviridae, Discoviridae, Fimoviridae, Hantaviridae, Leishbuviridae, Mypoviridae, Nairoviridae, Peribunyaviridae, Phasmaviridae, Phenuiviridae, Tospoviridae, Tulasviridae, and Wupedeviridae. Some viruses belonging to the order Bunyaviridaes can infect humans and lead to various disease syndromes, including febrile illness, encephalitis, hemorrhagic fever, and acute respiratory disease [2]. The family Tospoviridae is made up of viruses that only infect plants. Some bunyaviruses have a large impact on human health. For example, Crimean–Congo hemorrhagic fever (CCHF) occurs sporadically in many regions of Africa, Asia, and

Europe with a mortality rate of approximately 30% [3]. The main clinical manifestations of severe fever with thrombocytopenia syndrome (SFTS) caused by novel bunyavirus are high fever, thrombocytopenia, leukopenia, gastrointestinal symptoms, liver and kidney dysfunction, and even multiple organ dysfunction syndrome (MODS). Although LACV infection is rarely fatal (<1%), it may lead to long-term neurological sequelae such as seizures, hemiparesis, or cognitive/neurobehavioral abnormalities [4]. Due to the lack of specific antiviral treatments or vaccines, bunyavirus infections continue to pose a global threat to human health, affecting various populations in both developing and developed countries and potentially leading to outbreaks, which is a significant public health concern [5].

Interferon (IFN) is an important cytokine produced by the body when infected with viruses and can trigger antiviral immune responses. However, numerous studies show that a variety of bunyaviruses can inhibit IFN response, especially the type I IFN pathway [2]. Bunyaviruses evade the recognition and attack of the host by inhibiting IFN production and signal transduction to complete the initial replication and spread after successfully invading the host, which is closely related to the severity and death of the disease [6,7]. In recent years, researchers not only explored the mechanism of how bunyaviruses inhibit the signaling pathway of IFN production, but also revealed many key targets related to the regulation of IFN response that have potential prospects for antiviral drug development. In this paper, we review the current studies on the suppression of IFN response in bunyavirus infections. Furthermore, we summarize and predict the potential therapeutic approaches aiming at the key targets of IFN response that may be used for bunyavirus infections by countering the viral suppression of IFN responses.

2. Antiviral Effects of the IFN Response

IFN belongs to a family of cytokines that was first described in 1957 as the inhibitor of viral replication [8]. They not only play a role in various cancers and infections but also are capable of immunomodulation and have a major impact on the development and maintenance of innate and adaptive immunity [9–12]. IFN plays an essential role in the fight against various infections, especially as an anti-virus [13–18]. As a broad-spectrum antiviral agent, it inhibits both RNA and DNA viruses by inducing the expression of IFN-stimulated genes (ISGs). It mediates antiviral effects through viral RNA degradation, viral translation inhibition, or both. IFN can also directly activate immune cells and indirectly inhibit the replication process of viruses during early viral infections in the organism.

Based on the amino acid sequences of IFNs, they are categorized into three types, type I (IFNα, IFNβ, IFNδ, IFNε, IFNκ, IFNτ, IFNω, and IFNζ), type II (IFNγ), and type III (IFNλ) [19]. Among them, type I and type III IFNs are classic antiviral IFNs with highly similar reaction pathways. Type I IFNs have a protective effect in virus systemic infection, whereas the antiviral effect of type III IFNs is particularly pronounced at epithelial barriers such as the gastrointestinal, respiratory, and reproductive tracts [20,21]. Moreover, type I IFN response is rapid and strongly induced ISG production, while type III IFN induces a relatively slow and stable ISG response [22]. Unlike other IFNs, the main function of type II IFN is immunomodulatory and its antiviral effect is weak. However, it plays a special role in the long-term control of viral infection [13].

Type I IFNs have the largest number of family members, and the main subtypes studied are IFNα and IFNβ, which are also the most reported to play a role in antiviral responses. Type I IFNs are synthesized very rapidly because of the absence of introns in their gene structure and the few transcription factors they require [23]. Type I IFNs are produced mainly when PRRs on the cell surface or in the cytoplasm of most cell types are stimulated by PAMPs [24–26]. Among the PRRs are Toll-like receptors (TLRs), NOD-like receptors (NLRs), and RIG-like receptors (RLRs). In the TLR pathway, Toll/IL-1R domain-containing adaptor-inducing IFN-beta (TRIF) or myeloid differentiation factor-88 (MyD88) components are recruited to the activated receptor after the receptors receive a stimulus from viral ds/ss DNA/RNA [27]. Then, receptor-associated kinases such as TAK1 and tank-binding kinase 1 (TBK1) induce phosphorylation of key transcription factors such as

IFN regulatory factor 3 (IRF3), IFN regulatory factor 7 (IRF7), and nuclear factor kappa B (NF-κB), which are recruited to the promoter region of type I IFN genes to induce their transcriptions. In the RLR pathway, the retinoic acid-inducible gene (RIG-I), melanoma differentiation-associated protein 5 (MDA5), and laboratory of genetics and physiology 2 (LGP2) are activated after detecting viral RNA. LSm14A, a member of the LSm family, is a sensor of viral RNA and DNA that regulates the IFN response through RIG-I, which plays an important role in initiating IFN-β induction during the early stages of viral infection [28]. TRIM25 acts as an E3-ubiquitin ligase, whose RING structural domain interacts with RIG-I to mediate the caspase activation of RIG-I and interaction between its recruitment domain (CARD) and mitochondrial antiviral signaling protein (MAVS) [29]. RLR activates MAVS through aggregation, thereby activating IRF3, IRF7, and NF-κB, finally initiating type I IFN expression [30].

IFN then acts on specific cellular receptors to enhance the expression of hundreds of different genes collectively known as ISGs, including PKR, ISG15, ISG20, etc., thereby inducing an antiviral state [31–34]. Type I IFNs will bind to their specific receptors (a heterodimeric cell surface transmembrane receptor composed of IFNAR1 and IFNAR2 subunits) [35]. Then, the receptors rely on related Janus kinases (JAKs), such as TYK2 and JAK1 for signaling [35,36]. Activated JAKs phosphorylate specific tyrosine residues on the receptors, which dock with STAT1 and STAT2 [37], thereby phosphorylating them. Phosphorylated STAT1 and STAT2 bind to each other to form a stable heterodimer: the STAT1-STAT2 heterodimer. This dimer interacts with IRF9 to form the IRF9-STAT1-STAT2 heterodimer (ISGF3), which is translocated to the nucleus. ISGF3 induces the transcriptions of ISGs by activating the ISRE-containing promoter [38]. Additionally, type I IFNs and type II IFNs promote the formation of STAT1 dimer, termed the IFN-γ-activated factor (GAF), which is translocated to the nucleus and binds to the gamma-activated site (GAS) to induce ISGs expression [22,23,39].

Similar to type I IFNs, type III IFNs are induced by viral-derived PAMPs, but the molecular mechanism is not yet clear [39]. Induction of type III IFNs by the RLRs pathway is similar to that of type I IFNs. Different from type I IFNs, MAVS can be recruited to peroxisome and mitochondria, which is recruited to peroxisome and induces type III IFNs preferentially [40]. Type III IFNs have a similar signaling pattern to type I IFNs [41], which is achieved by binding to their receptor complexes, and signaling also occurs through the JAK-STAT signaling pathway. The receptor complexes consist of cell surface-specific IFNLR1 and IL-10R2 (Figure 1) [42].

IFN-γ is the sole member of type II IFN, which is produced primarily by antigen-activated T cells and NK cells. Additionally, macrophages secrete it under certain circumstances [43,44]. The antiviral effect of IFN-γ mostly relies on PKR, adenosine deaminase RNA specific-1 (ADAR-1), interferon-induced transmembrane proteins (IFITMs), and tripartite motif-containing proteins (TRIMs) that are induced by IFN-γ [45]. IFN-γ is induced by mitogens and cytokines such as IL-12, IL-15, IL-18, IL-27, and type I IFNs [46,47]. JAKs are activated when these cytokines bind to corresponding cell surface receptors, which in turn phosphorylates and activates STATs. Subsequently, the production and secretion of IFN-γ are promoted [47,48]. These STATs may be STAT1, STAT3, STAT4, or STAT5 [47]. The signaling pattern of type II IFNs is similar to type I IFNs and type III IFNs. The IFNGR complex is the type II IFN receptor. The difference is that IFN-γ signaling mainly activates GAF that targets GAS DNA sequences. Furthermore, IFN-γ also can activate ISGF3 [22,23,39] (Figure 1).

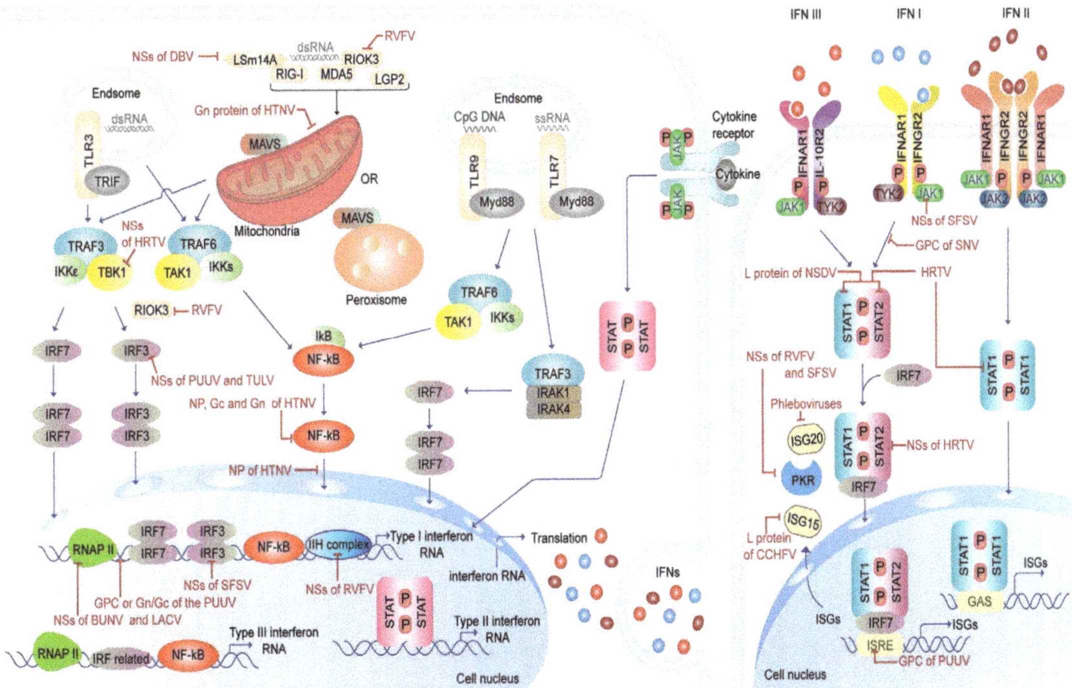

Figure 1. Anti-viral IFN response pathways and known suppression mechanisms of it in the order Bunyavirales.

A. After virus invasion, the IFN pathway is activated to play an antiviral role. IFNs are categorized into three types, type I, type II, and type III. The PRRs include Toll-like receptors (TLRs), NOD-like receptors (NLRs), and RIG-like receptors (RLRs). In the TLR pathway, viral ds/ss DNA/RNA is recognized by TLRs on the endosome after the virus is broken down in the endosome. Then Toll/IL-1R domain-containing adaptor-inducing IFN-beta (TRIF) or myeloid differentiation factor-88 (MyD88) are recruited to the TLRs. TAK1 and TBK1 are activated to induce phosphorylation of IFN regulatory factor 3 (IRF3), IFN regulatory factor 7 (IRF7), and nuclear factor kappa B (NF-κB), which are recruited to the promoter region of type I IFN genes to induce their transcriptions. In the RLR pathway, the retinoic acid-inducible gene (RIG-I), melanoma differentiation-associated protein 5 (MDA5), and laboratory of genetics and physiology 2 (LGP2) are activated after detecting viral RNA. RLR activates mitochondrial antiviral signaling protein (MAVS) through aggregation, thereby activating IRF3, IRF7, and NF-κB, finally initiating type I IFN expression. LSm14A, a sensor of viral RNA and DNA, regulates the IFN response through RIG-I. TRIM25 interacts with RIG-I to mediate the activation of RIG-I and the interaction between RIG-I and MAVS. The generated type I IFNs will bind to their specific receptors. Then the receptors rely on related Janus kinases (JAKs), such as TYK2 and JAK1 for signaling, activated JAKs phosphorylate specific tyrosine residues on the receptors, which dock with STAT1 and STAT2, make them phosphorylated, and form a stable STAT1-STAT2 heterodimer. This dimer interacts with IRF9 to form the IRF9-STAT1-STAT2 heterodimer (ISGF3), which is translocated to the nucleus to induce the transcriptions of IFN-stimulated genes (ISGs) by activating the IFN-stimulated response element (ISRE)-containing promoter. Additionally, type I IFNs and type II IFNs promote the formation of STAT1 dimer, termed IFN-γ-activated factor (GAF), which is translocated to the nucleus and binds to the gamma-activated site (GAS) to induce ISGs expression. Cytokines can bind to corresponding cell surface receptors, make JAKs phosphorylation and activate STATs, then promote the production and secretion of type II IFN. The signaling pattern of type II IFNs is similar to type I IFNs. The differences are that the IFNGR is the type II IFN receptor and IFN-γ signaling mainly activates GAF that targets GAS. Induction of type III IFNs by the RLRs pathway is similar to that of type I IFNs. The difference is that MAVS can be recruited to peroxisome and mitochondria, which is recruited to peroxisome and induces type III IFNs preferentially. Type III IFNs have a similar signaling pattern to type I IFNs, achieved by binding to their receptor complexes (FNLR1 and IL-10R2).

B. In the interferon-producing pathway, viruses can act at different nodes to inhibit the antiviral effect of interferon. NSs of Dabie bandavirus (DBV) can interact and co-localize with LSm14A to inhibit the activation of RIG-I to reduce IRF3 phosphorylation and dimerization. Rift Valley fever virus (RVFV) can induce alternative splicing of RIOK3 transcript and then attenuate IFN response. Gn protein of hantaan virus (HTNV) can translocate to mitochondria and interact with mitochondrial Tu translation elongation factor (TUFM) to recruit LC3B and degrade MAVS. NSs of heartland virus (HRTV) can interact with TBK1 to block the binding of TBK1 to IRF3, thus inhibiting type I IFN induction. NSs of Puumala virus (PUUV)/Tula virus (TULV) can inhibit downstream factor IRF3 activity and IFN-β promoter. High-dose NP, Gc, and Gn of HTNV can inhibit NF-κB activation and interferon-stimulated gene expression and NP can sequester NF-κB in the cytoplasm and inhibit the activity of NF-κB. Bunyamwera orthobunyavirus (BUNV) NSs interact with MED8 to prevent the phosphorylation of RNA polymerase II (RNAP II). La Crosse virus (LACV) NSs degrade the IIo-borne RBP1 subunits by exploiting the cellular DNA damage. GPC or Gn/Gc of PUUV can inhibit the activation of IFN-β promoter. Sandfly fever Sicilian virus (SFSV) NSs can inhibit the induction of IFN by shielding the DNA-binding domain of IRF3. RVFV NSs can interfere with the formation of the transcription factor IIH complex. SFSV NSs can directly interact with JAK1 to inhibit STAT1 phosphorylation. GPC of Sin Nombre virus (SNV) can strongly inhibit the induction of IFN-β and the downstream amplification of the JAK-STAT pathway. The L protein of the Nairobi sheep disease virus (NSDV) can inhibit the phosphorylation of STAT1 and STAT2. HRTV can directly inhibit STAT1 without the help of viral protein and its NSs can interact and colocalize with STAT2 to specifically block the nuclear translocation of STAT2. RVFV NSs can trigger degradation of PKR and SFSV NSs can bind to eIF2B and maintain eIF2B activity against translational inhibition caused by PKR. Phleboviruses can largely escape the antiviral effect of ISG20. The L protein of Crimean–Congo hemorrhagic fever virus (CCHFV) can reduce ISG15-encoded ubiquitin and the conjugation of ubiquitin-like proteins with cellular proteins. GPC of PUUV can antagonize the promoter of ISRE on ISGs.

3. Suppressing IFN Response Mechanisms of Bunyavirales

The order Bunyavirales consists of RNA viruses, including more than 500 different viruses and strains, which are classified into fourteen families. These viruses utilize host cell proteins to facilitate their replication and transcription. The viral invasion of host cells enhances the transcriptional level of IFN, NF-κB, and inflammasome signaling pathways, inducing the expression of a large number of pro-inflammatory cytokines, and finally initiating the host antiviral innate immune response, the IFN response. The virulence of pathogenic bunyaviruses is directly related to the actions of viral virulence factors and their ability to counteract host immunity. Arthropod-borne viruses are distributed worldwide. Although some remain unnoticed or are associated with mild flu-like symptoms, many are significant human and veterinary pathogens that cause severe diseases such as arthritis, gastroenteritis, encephalitis, hemorrhagic fever, etc. Moreover, they lead to devastating economic losses due to reduced livestock productivity and high mortality rates. RNA gene segments of different bunyaviruses are heterogeneous, but most of them share similar characteristic molecular structures; that is, the presence of viral nonstructural proteins as interferon antagonists. In this context, we mainly discuss the strategies employed by bunyaviruses to evade the antiviral state induced by IFN in infected cells.

DBV is a novel kind of bunyavirus. The IFN inhibitory response of DBV is primarily mediated by NSs and cytoplasmic structures called viral inclusion bodies (IBs) that they induce. NSs can directly interact with signaling molecules such as TRIM25, TBK1, Ikk, IRF7, and STAT2, and sequester them into the viral IBs, thereby inhibiting the IFN response. NS protein interacts with TRIM25 and tethers it to the viral IBs in order to inhibit TRIM25-mediated RIG-I-Ly-63-linked ubiquitination or activation, thus suppressing RLR-mediated antiviral signaling and IFN gene expression [49,50]. DBV NSs can effectively capture TBK1 and IKKε to IBs, interfering with TBK1/IKKε-IRF3/IRF7 signaling, which is closely associated with the amino acids serine 21 and leucine 23 in NSs [51,52]. DBV NSs can also sequester IRF7 and STAT2, but not STAT1 to IBs, thereby preventing STAT2 phosphorylation and nuclear translocation, eventually blocking type I IFN-stimulated JAK-STAT signaling and inhibiting the expression of ISGs [53,54]. However, there is a study showing that NSs can isolate both into viral IBs to impair STAT2 phosphorylation induced by IFN and the nuclear translocation of both STATs, leading to inhibition of the IFN-JAK-STAT signaling pathway and ISGs expression [55] (Figure 2). Additionally, LSm14A plays an important role in the early induction of IFN-beta during virus infection. Nevertheless, DBV NSs effectively inhibit IRF3 phosphorylation and dimerization by interacting and co-localizing with LSm14A. The second arginine in the conserved leucine-rich repeat domain (LRRD) at the N-terminus of NSs is crucial for its interaction with LSm14A [56].

Guertu virus (GTV) is a newly isolated potential highly pathogenic bunyavirus in China, with genetic relation to DBV and HRTV. In terms of GTV, its cytoplasmic structures antagonizing IFN response differ from DBV. GTV NSs (G-NSs) induce the formation of dense IBs and filamentous structures (FSs) in the cytoplasm. G-NSs interact with TBK1 and STAT2, thereby irreversibly isolating them into the viral IBs and FSs, finally inhibiting the phosphorylation, activation, and nuclear translocation of IRF3 [57] (Figure 2).

HRTV is a recently reclassified member of the genus Bandavirus, family Phenuiviridae of order Bunyavirales. Likewise, HRTV can antagonize the host's innate immune response. However, it does not encode any viral protein but acts as a direct antagonist against STAT1, and it can reduce the activation of STAT2 and STAT1 induced by type I and type III IFNs excluding IFNγ [58]. The similarity in the mechanism of IFN response antagonism between HRTV and DBV lies in the fact that the NSs of both viruses can interact with TBK1 and then hinder the binding of TBK1 to its substrate IRF3, thus blocking IRF3 activation and cellular transcriptional induction, which depends on two conserved amino acids at positions 21 and 23 [52,59]. Additionally, both viral NS proteins can interact with STAT2 to prevent its nuclear translocation. The difference is that HRTV NSs do not interact with STAT1 and do not affect the nuclear translocation of STAT1 [58]. Yet now there is no research indicating that HRTV NSs can induce unique cytoplasmic structures such as viral inclusion bodies and filamentous structures.

Similar to DBV, GTV, and HRTV, Nairobi sheep disease virus (NSDV) can also inhibit the production of IFN by interfering with STAT1 and STAT2. NSDV is another member of the genus Orthonairovirus in the family Nairoviridae, which is a tick-borne zoonotic pathogen genetically related to the human-pathogenic CCHFV. NSDV can lead to severe and often fatal hemorrhagic gastroenteritis. There is evidence that the L protein of NSDV can inhibit the phosphorylation of STAT1 and STAT2 in Vero cells, particularly in response to I and II type IFN stimulation, with STAT1 being the primary target and this inhibitory effect is related to the enzymatic activity of the N-terminal OTU domain of the L protein [60].

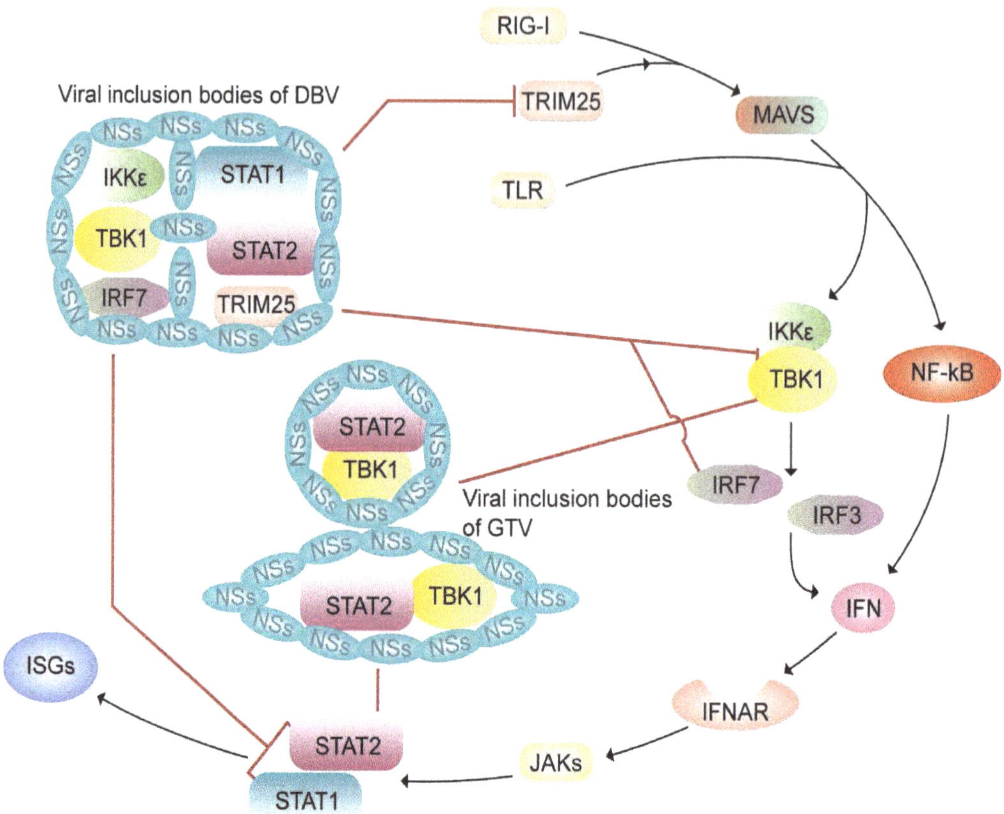

Figure 2. Model for DBV and GTV suppressing the IFN antiviral system by NS sequestration of key signaling molecules into IBs or FSs. After Dabie bandavirus (DBV) invades the host cells, TRIM25, tank-binding kinase 1 (TBK1), Ikkε, IFN regulatory factor 7 (IRF7), and STAT2, which are involved in the IFN signaling pathway, interact with DBV NSs and are captured into inclusion bodies (IBs), thereby inhibiting the IFN signaling pathway. TRIM25 is isolated to the viral IBs to inhibit TRIM25-mediated retinoic acid-inducible gene (RIG-I)-Ly-63-linked ubiquitination or activation. Reduction in intracellular free TBK1 and IKKε interferes with TBK1/IKKε- IFN regulatory factor 3 (IRF3)/IRF7 signaling. DBV NSs prevent the nuclear translocation of IRF7 by sequestering it to IBs. The phosphorylation and nuclear translocation of STAT2 are inhibited by IBs, which block type I IFN-stimulated JAK-STAT signaling. STAT1 may be tethered to the viral IBs that block its nuclear translocation, resulting in the inhibition of IFN signaling and IFN-stimulated genes (ISGs) expression. Likewise, NSs of Guertu virus (GTV) hijack TBK1 and STAT2 into IBs and filamentous structures (FSs) affecting the corresponding signal transduction.

Rift Valley fever virus (RVFV) is also a member of the order Bunyavirales, belonging to the Phlebovirus genus, family Phenuiviridae. It caused periodic outbreaks in livestock and humans in African and Middle Eastern countries. RVFV NS is a major virulence factor that disrupts the host-innate immune response and antagonizes IFN [61]. The NSs protein of RVFV can inhibit the transcription of type I IFN-β gene, but strains with intact NS protein can still activate the dimerization and nuclear translocation of RIG-I, IRF3, and nuclear translocation of NF-κB, which suggests that NSs protein inhibits the up-regulation of downstream IFN-β promoters activated by transcription factors to evade host innate immunity [62]. RVFV NSs can interact with two transcription factors, SAP30 and YY1, that regulate IFN-β to interfere with the formation of the transcription factor IIH complex, degrade the p62 subunit, and sequester the p44 subunit, which finally suppresses the host's IFN-β gene transcription and can trigger specific degradation of PKR through proteasomal degradation [63–65]. A significant portion of the antiviral activity of IFN against RVFV was attributed to PKR. The NSs can induce the degradation of PKR, thereby preventing the phosphorylation of eIF2α in cells, allowing the virus to efficiently translate and replicate [66]. RIO kinase 3 (RIOK3) is a protein kinase that facilitates the activation of MDA5 and IRF3 in the process of IFN-β production [67,68]. Experiments show that RVFV infection induces selective splicing of the RIOK3 transcript, which weakens the IFN response [69]. Furthermore, Barski proposed that the filament arrangement of the NS's core structural domain in the crystal may reveal the molecular basis of how the virulence factor NS assembles in the cell nucleus, which is crucial for a fundamental understanding of RVFV's interference with the IFN immune response [70].

The NSs of Sandfly fever Sicilian virus (SFSV) play an important role in suppressing interferon responses. The SFSV can not only inhibit IRF3 and JAK-STAT pathway, but also inhibit PKR as RVFV. SFSV is one of the most common members of the genus Phlebovirus, family Phenuiviridae. Its NSs can inhibit IFN induction by blocking the IRF3 DNA-binding domain, thereby interfering with the RIG-I-TBK1-IRF3 signaling pathway [71]. SFSV NSs can also directly interact with JAK1 to inhibit STAT1 phosphorylation and nuclear translocation, thereby suppressing the signal transduction of the type I IFN [72]. Its NSs tightly bind to eIF2B to block the binding of eIF2-p to eIF2B, thereby maintaining the activity of eIF2B to prevent translation inhibition caused by PKR, eventually maintaining the synthesis of viral proteins [73].

Hantaan virus (HTNV) not only acts on NF-κB similar to RVFV but also acts on MAVS to suppress IFN. Moreover, the glycoprotein N (Gn) and nucleocapsid protein (NP) of HTNV play an essential role in IFN suppression. HTNV is the pathogen responsible for Korean hemorrhagic fever, which belongs to the orthohantavirus genus (order Bunyavirales, family Hantaviridae). HTNV can induce hemorrhagic fever with renal syndrome characterized by endothelial dysfunction, as well as hantavirus pulmonary syndrome, both of which have high fatality rates. HTNV infection can suppress the antiviral effects of all IFNs (including type III IFN). NP can sequester NF-κB in the cytoplasm, inhibiting tumor necrosis factor-alpha (TNF-α) and interfering with host innate immune responses [74]. Additionally, NP can enhance the activity of the miR-146a promoter, promoting miR-146a expression and its negative regulatory effect on the NF-κB pathway [75]. At high doses, both NP and envelope proteins (Gn and Gc) can inhibit NF-κB activation and the expression of IFN-stimulated genes, thus suppressing the IFN response [76]. In the early stages of infection, HTNV induces complete mitophagy, followed by incomplete mitophagy in later stages and these responses involve the viral Gn and NP. The viral Gn in infected cells can translocate to the mitochondria and interact with TUFM, promoting mitophagy by recruiting LC3B. Then the degradation of MAVS is promoted, finally suppressing the type I IFN response. The viral NP competes with Gn for binding to LC3B and interacts with SNAP29 to disturb the autophagic degradation of Gn [77]. Consequently, both Gn and NP of HTNV can inhibit IFN response by degrading MAVS.

Puumala virus (PUUV), Tula virus (TULV), and Sin Nombre virus (SNV) are the other three members of the orthohantavirus genus (order Bunyavirales, family Hantaviridae). The glycoprotein precursor (GPC) is important for the IFN suppression of them. The GPC or its cleavage product Gn/Gc of PUUV can inhibit the activation of IFN-β promoter triggered by RIG-I. Furthermore, the GPC of PUUV and TULV can antagonize the promoter of IFN-stimulated response element (ISRE) on ISGs [78]. Likewise, the GPC of SNV strongly inhibits IFN-β induction and signaling transduction by suppressing downstream signaling of the JAK-STAT pathway [79]. The functional NSs of both PUUV and TULV can inhibit the activity of downstream factor IRF3 and IFN-β promoter [80].

The similarity between Bunyamwera orthobunyavirus (BUNV) and LACV lies in that the NSs of both can suppress the induction of IFN by affecting RNAP II. BUNV is the prototype of the genus orthobunyavirus (Bunyavirales: Peribunyaviridae), which poses a significant threat to human health and food security. LACV is the major cause of pediatric arboviral encephalitis in the United States and LACV encephalitis can result in learning and memory impairments, with over 80% of reported cases of neurological diseases occurring in children. The N-terminal and C-terminal regions of BUNV NSs play a critical role in countering the host antiviral response [81–83]. The C-terminal region of BUNV NSs interacts with cellular mediator protein MED8 to prevent the phosphorylation of serine 2 in the C-terminal domain (CTD) of RNAP II, thereby interfering with IFN synthesis of the mammalian host [82]. NSs from BUNV and RVFV interact with two host cell factors, MED8 and p44, to inhibit RNAP II. However, LACV NSs employ a distinct mechanism to inhibit or degrade RNAP II. In LACV-infected cells, NSs degrade the IIo-borne RBP1 subunits by exploiting the cellular DNA damage response pathway [84]. Research suggested that the E3 ubiquitin ligase elongin C subunit of LACV acts as an NS co-factor in RBP1 degradation to block RIG-I-induced IFN production and inhibit the synthesis of IFN-related mRNA [85]. Tacaiuma virus (TCMV), another member of the genus Orthobunyavirus in the family Peribunyaviridae, causes an acute febrile illness accompanied by muscle and joint pain [86], whose pathogenic mechanism does not involve NSs.

ISG20 and ISG15 are the other two key points of IFN suppression in some members of the order Bunyavirales infections. ISG20 is an anti-bunyavirus factor, and its anti-bunyavirus activity depends on its functional RNase activity. ISG20 has strong antiviral activity against most viruses from the Peribunyaviridae, Hantavirus, and Nairovirus genera, but it does not affect Phleboviruses [87]. This suggests that the ability of Phleboviruses to escape ISG20 may affect their pathogenesis. CCHFV belongs to the genus Orthonairovirus in the family Nairoviridae of the order Bunyavirales. Earlier research discovered that the L protein of CCHFV reduces ISG15-encoded ubiquitin and the conjugation of ubiquitin-like proteins with cellular proteins, and then interferes with IFN induction, which is related to the N-terminal OTU domain of the L protein [60]. Meanwhile, there is evidence that the NSDV negatively regulates the IFN induction by encoding an OTU family protease [88].

In summary, host cells can sense viral infections and activate the innate immune system to inhibit viral replication and propagation. When PAMPs are recognized by PRRs within cells, numerous signaling cascades are activated, thereby leading to the production of IFNs. IFNs establish an antiviral state by inducing the expression of hundreds of ISGs in an autocrine and/or paracrine manner. The IFN response induced after bunyavirus infections can restrict the infection at various steps of the viral life cycle, including viral entry, genome transcription and replication, and viral particle exocytosis. The main processes of the IFN response include TLR-dependent signaling, MDA5 and RIG-I-dependent signaling, IFN antiviral signaling transduction, and IFN-inducible transcriptions. Bunyaviruses can counteract this antiviral response by avoiding cellular recognition of PAMPs, inhibiting IFN production, or interfering with IFN-mediated antiviral responses (Figures 1 and 2). Furthermore, the key targets involved in this counteraction include RLRs, TBK1, IRF3, and JAK, among other immune molecules (Table 1). Therefore, it may serve as a potential measure in the treatment of bunyavirus infections to target directly or indirectly these key immune molecules.

Table 1. The current research status of the suppressing interferon response mechanisms in Bunyavirales.

Viral Name	Main Targets/ Pathways	Mechanisms for the Suppression of IFN Response	Relevant Amino Acid Sites	References
DBV	TRIM25	NSs → IBs → sequester TRIM25 → RIG-I activity ↓	\	[49,50]
	TBK1, IKKε	NSs → IBs → sequester TBK1 and IKKε → TBK1/IKKε-IRF3/IRF7 signaling ↓	Amino acids serine 21 and leucine 23 in NSs.	[51,52]
	IRF7	NSs → IBs → nuclear translocation of IRF7 ↓	\	[54]
	STAT2	NSs → IBs → sequester STAT2, but not STAT1 → phosphorylation and nuclear translocation of STAT2 ↓	\	[53]
	STAT1, STAT2	NSs → IBs → sequester STAT2 and STAT1 → phosphorylation of STAT2 ↓, nuclear translocations of STAT2 ↓ and STAT1 ↓	\	[55]
	LSm14A	NSs → LSm14A → RIG-I activity ↓	The second arginine in the LRRD at the N-terminus of NSs.	[56]
GTV	TBK1, STAT2	NSs → IBs, FSs → sequester TBK1 and STAT2	\	[57]
HRTV	TBK1	NSs → TBK1 → IRF3 activity ↓	Amino acids serine 21 and leucine 23 in NSs.	[52,59]
	STAT1	Without the help of viral protein → STAT1 ↓	\	[58]
	STAT2	NSs → STAT2 → nuclear translocation of STAT2 ↓	\	[58]
NSDV	STAT1, STAT2	L protein → phosphorylation of STAT1 ↓ and STAT2 ↓	\	[60]
RVFV	Transcription factor IIH complex, PKR	NSs → SAP30, YY1 → transcription factor IIH complex ↓, PKR ↓	\	[63–65]
	RIOK3	Viral infection → RIOK3 ↓	\	[69]
SFSV	IRF3	NSs → shield the DNA-binding domain of IRF3 → TBK1-IRF3 ↓	\	[71]
	JAK1	NSs → JAK1 → phosphorylation and nuclear translocation of STAT1 ↓ in type I IFN response	\	[72]
	PKR	NSs → eIF2B activity ↑ → translational inhibition effect of PKR ↓	\	[73]
HTNV	MAVS	Gn → TUFM → degrade MAVS	\	[77]
	NF-κB	NP → sequester NF-κB in the cytoplasm, NF-κB activity ↓	\	[74]
	NF-κB	NP → miR-146a ↑ → NF-κB pathway ↓	\	[75]
	NF-κB	NP, Gn, Gc → NF-κB activity ↓, ISGs expression ↓	\	[76]
PUUV	\	GPC, Gn/Gc → IFN-β promoter activity ↓	\	[78]
	ISRE	GPC → antagonizes ISRE on ISGs	\	[78]
	IRF3	NSs → IRF3 activity ↓, IFN-β promoter activity ↓	\	[80]
TULV	IRF3	NSs → IRF3 activity ↓, IFN-β promoter activity ↓	\	[80]
SNV	JAK-STAT	GPC → JAK-STAT ↓	\	[79]
BUNV	RNAP II	NSs → MED8, p44 → dysregulate RNAP II	\	[82]

Table 1. *Cont.*

Viral Name	Main Targets/ Pathways	Mechanisms for the Suppression of IFN Response	Relevant Amino Acid Sites	References
LACV	RNAP II	NSs → DNA damage response pathway → degrade IIo-borne RBP1 subunits → RNAP II ↓ NSs and cofactor Elongin C → degrade RNAP II subunit RPB1 → RNAP II ↓	\	[84,85]
Phleboviruses	ISG20	Escape the antiviral effect of ISG20	\	[87]
CCHFV	ISG15	L protein → ISG15-encoded ubiquitin ↓, the conjugation of ubiquitin-like proteins with cellular proteins ↓	\	[60]

Note: \ No research indicated amino acid sites of viral proteins associated with the corresponding IFN suppression mechanism; DBV, Dabie bandavirus; GTV, Guertu virus; HRTV, Heartland virus; NSDV, Nairobi sheep disease virus; BUNV, Bunyamwera orthobunyavirus; LACV, La Crosse encephalitis virus; RVFV, Rift Valley fever virus; SFSV, Sandfly fever Sicilian virus; HTNV, Hantaan virus; PUUV, Puumala virus; TULV, Tula virus; SNV, Sin Nombre virus; CCHFV, Crimean–Congo hemorrhagic fever virus; RNAP II, RNA polymerase II; ISRE, IFN-stimulated response element; NSs, the non-structural proteins; PKR, protein kinase R; RIOK3, RIO kinase 3; MED8, mediator complex subunit 8; RBP1, retinol-binding protein type 1; TUFM, mitochondrial Tu translation elongation factor; LC3B, noncanonical light chain 3B; Gn, glycoprotein n; NP, nucleocapsid protein; Gc, glycoprotein C; GPC, glycoprotein precursor; ISGs, IFN-stimulated genes; IBs, inclusion bodies; FSs, filamentous structures; SAP30, Sin3A-associated protein 30; YY1, Yin Yang 1, an oncogenic transcription factor; and LRRD, leucine-rich repeat domain.

4. Potential Treatment Options for IFN Suppression

IFN response plays a crucial role in the development of various diseases, and numerous studies explored the impact of regulating its key targets on diseases. Some of these studies were already applied clinically in antiviral treatments. However, in terms of bunyavirus infections, specific therapeutic research is lacking. Nevertheless, certain drugs, compounds, or methods associated with IFN response regulation might possess potential antiviral effects against bunyaviruses, which are expected to be used in the treatment of bunyavirus infections. Based on the key IFN pathway nodes and viral proteins of the suppression of IFN response in bunyavirus infections, this article reviews drugs, compounds, and methods closely related to their regulation and analyzes their clinical applications, particularly in the context of virus infections (Table 2). These treatments directly or indirectly influence IFN response and its antiviral signaling, representing potential therapeutic strategies for bunyavirus infections.

Table 2. Antiviral research and potential strategies based on key targets of IFN response pathways and viral proteins.

Key Targets	Potential Strategies against Bunyavirus	Research and Applications of Antiviral Therapy	Reference
	RLR		
RIG-I and MDA5	PolyI: C; BO-112 MSCs	Mengo virus, RSV, SARS-CoV-2 HIV, HBV, SARS-CoV-2	[89–92] [93–98]
RIG-I	NTZ	Influenza virus, Viral gastroenteritis, RV, EBOV	[99–102]
	Acitretin	HIV, BKPyV, HPV	[103–105]
	Salidroside	DENV, CVB3, IAV	[106–109]
	RNA agonists of RIG-I: 3p10LG9, 5′-pppRNA, 5′-ppp siRNA, 3p-siRNA-MDR1, and SLR14	IAV, DENV, HSV-1, SARS-CoV-2	[110–115]
	IR; DNA-damaging agents: doxorubicin, etoposide, teniposide, and oxaliplatin	ZIKV, Influenza virus, Poliovirus, SARS-CoV-2, DENV	[116–122]

Table 2. *Cont.*

Key Targets	Potential Strategies Against Bunyavirus	Research and Applications of Antiviral Therapy	Reference
MDA5	DNA demethylation agents: DNMTis such as AZA and DAC	\	[123–125]
TBK1	Lidocaine	IAV, SARS-CoV-2	[126]
IRF3	Isoflavone and isoflavone-like compounds: KIN 101, genistein	HCV, Influenza virus, AdV, HSV, HIV, RV	[127,128]
	Hydroxyquinoline family compounds: KIN1400, KIN1408, KIN1409	WNV, DENV, HCV, IAV, RSV, NiV, LASV, EBOV	[129]
Others	P97 inhibitors: clotrimazole	Poliovirus, HSV, CMV, Influenza virus	[130,131]
	ERRα inverse agonist: XCT790; ERRα inhibitors: compound A, kaempferol, compound B, LingH2-10, naringenin, SR16388, five anticancer drugs and nine pesticides that inhibit ERRα activity	CMV, VSV, NDV, HSV, HBV	[132–141]
	7-DHC; DHCR7 inhibitors: tamoxifen, AY9944, haloperidol, aripiprazole, cariprazine, trazodone, BM15.766	ZIKV, VSV, HCV, HSV, SARS-CoV-2	[142–150]
	SOCS antagonist: pJAK2 (1001–1013)	HSV-1, IAV, VV, EMCV, DENV, ZIKV, WNV, EBOV	[151–154]
	MEKi: trametinib	IAV, RV2, RSVA2	[155–157]
NSs	RNAi	RVFV, IAV, PRRSV, WNV, SARS-CoV-2	[158–162]
NP	doxycycline and minocycline	CCHFV	[163]
	curcumin	IAV, EBOV, HIV, DENV, HSV-2, etc.	[164–166]
	naproxen	IAV, SARS-CoV-2	[167,168]
	compound RK424	IAV	[169]
	RNAi	hMPV, RABV, BoDV-1, IAV	[170–173]
	NP-specific mAbs	IAV	[174]
	antisense oligonucleotides	AIV H5N1	[175]
GPC	trametinib	LUJV	[176]
Gn	2-DG	LCMV, SARS-CoV-2, HPV18, RV, HBV, HSV, etc.	[177,178]

Note: \, No research; MSCs, mesenchymal stromal cells; NTZ, nitazoxanide; IR, ionizing radiation; DNMTis, DNA methyltransferase inhibitors; AZA, 5-azacytidine; DAC, 5-aza-2′-deoxycytidine; compound A, N-[(2Z)-3-(4,5-dihydro-1,3-thiazol-2-yl)-1,3-thiazolidin-2-ylidene]-5H dibenzo[a,-d] [7]annulen-5-amine; compound B, cyclohexylmethyl-(1-p-tolyl-1H-indol-3-ylmethyl)-amine; 7-DHC, 7-dehydrocholesterol; DHCR7, 7-dehydrocholesterol reductase; MEKi, MEK inhibitor; RNAi, RNA interference; 2-DG, 2-deoxy-D-glucose; RSV, respiratory syncytial virus; HBV, hepatitis B virus; RV, rotavirus; EBOV, Ebola virus; BKPyV, BK polyomavirus; HPV, human papillomavirus; CVB3, coxsackievirus B3; IAV, influenza A virus; DENV, dengue virus; HSV-1, herpes simplex virus 1; ZIKV, zika virus; HCV, hepatitis C virus; HSV, herpes simplex virus; AdV, adenovirus; WNV, West Nile virus; NiV, Nipah virus; LASV, Lassa virus; PRRSV, porcine reproductive and respiratory syndrome virus; VSV, vesicular stomatitis virus; RV2, respiratory viruses rhinovirus; RSVA2, respiratory syncytial virus; CMV, cytomegalovirus; NDV, newcastle disease virus; VV, vaccinia virus; EMCV, encephalomyocarditis virus, CCHFV, Crimean–Congo hemorrhagic fever virus; hMPV, human metapneumovirus; RABV, rabies virus; BoDV-1, Borna disease virus; AIV, avian influenza virus; LUJV, Lujo virus; LCMV, lymphocytic choriomeningitis virus; and RV, rhinoviruses.

4.1. Key Targets of the IFN Pathway

4.1.1. RLR

RLRs are crucial sensors in viral infections and important inducers of type I IFNs and other antiviral immune mediators. This protein family includes three members: RIG-I, MDA5, and LGP2. Among these, RIG-I and MDA5 are important inducers of type I IFN [179]. However, some viruses within the order Bunyavirales, such as DBV and RVFV, can suppress the IFN induction by impacting their activity. There are experimental and clinical studies showing that RLRs can be activated by synthetic RNA, oncolytic viruses, viral mimicry, and radiochemotherapy, leading to the expression of RLR-mediated IFNs and ISGs [180], which is essential for antiviral immunity in the host.

RIG-I and MDA5

Polyinosinic-polycytidylic acid (polyI:C) is a synthetic analog of double-stranded RNA as a viral mimic, which also is an agonist for TLR3 and RLR. It enhances RLR signaling, thereby strengthening RLR-mediated IFN responses to exhibit antiviral effects. Research demonstrated that polyI:C-induced IFN responses have a protective effect against mouse Mengo virus infection [89]. Furthermore, a recombinant trimeric spike protein vaccine containing PIKA, a stabilized derivative of polyI:C, as an adjuvant was proven to be effective against COVID-19 [91]. Another vaccine formulation containing polyI:C, innate defense regulator peptide, and polyphosphazine (ΔF/TriAdj) effectively immunizes newborns against respiratory syncytial virus (RSV) [92]. Thus, polyI:C might be a vital potential therapeutic compound and vaccine adjuvant for bunyaviruses. BO-112, a nanocomposite formulation of Poly I:C, and polyethyleneimine, can induce apoptosis in tumor cells displaying immunogenic cell death features [90]. It is capable of stimulating IFN response by polyI:C, thereby exerting its antiviral effects.

Mesenchymal stromal cells (MSCs) derived from bone marrow (BM), adipose tissue (AT), Wharton's jelly (WJ), and foreskin (FSK) have functional RIG-I and MDA-5 receptors. Upon receptor activation, IFN production is induced through TBK1/IKK-ε and IRF7 phosphorylation. Consequently, IFN's antiviral immune protective effect is enhanced [94]. Currently, MSCs made significant breakthroughs in addressing hematologic disorders, cardiovascular diseases, cirrhosis, neurological disorders, partial meniscectomy injury repair, and autoimmune diseases [93,95]. There are numerous completed or ongoing clinical trials exploring MSCs' preventive or therapeutic effects against HIV and hepatitis B virus (HBV) infections [97]. A series of phase 2 clinical trials showed that MSCs can be used to treat patients with severe COVID-19 patients [96,98]. Notably, MSCs can enhance virus-induced IFN responses, and are widely used in clinical antiviral treatment research, showing potential in bunyavirus infections treatment.

RIG-I

The U.S. Food and Drug Administration (FDA)-approved oral drug nitazoxanide (NTZ) targeting RIG-I and antiviral phosphatases GADD34 can increase the activities of RLR, mitochondrial antiviral signaling protein, IRF3, and IFN, which can also induce the transcription of GADD34 [101]. Currently, nitazoxanide is FDA-approved for the treatment of diarrhea caused by Cryptosporidium infection and is well-tolerated. Additionally, clinical trials indicated that NTZ reduces the duration of symptoms for influenza [100], viral gastroenteritis [102], and rotavirus (RV)-induced diarrhea [99]. It is also a potential oral therapy for the Ebola virus (EBOV) [101]. Nitazoxanide can enhance IFN antiviral immune responses, finally exhibiting antiviral effects, which represents a potential drug for treating bunyavirus infections.

Another drug approved by the FDA is acitretin, which induces RIG-I expression and enhances RIG-I signaling in vitro, thereby stimulating RIG-I-dependent IFN cascade reactions and inducing preferential apoptosis of HIV-infected cells. It is a potential drug to eliminate reactivating cells in latent HIV reservoirs [104]. Research showed that acitretin selectively inhibits BK polyomavirus (BKPyV) replication in primary human cells in nephropathy and hemorrhagic cystitis [103]. Combined immunotherapy using systemic acitretin and diphenylcyclopropenone effectively treats recalcitrant viral warts caused by human papillomavirus (HPV) infections [105]. Acitretin promotes RIG-I-dependent IFN response and antiviral effects. Therefore, acitretin might be a potential drug for treating bunyavirus infections in the future.

Salidroside is a prolyl endopeptidase inhibitor that exerts antiviral activity against dengue virus (DENV) by increasing the expression of RIG-I, thereby enhancing downstream signal cascades such as upregulation of IRF-3 and IRF-7, eventually stimulating IFN-mediated innate antiviral immunity. Additionally, it inhibits virus protein synthesis by increasing the expression of PKR and P-eIF2α while suppressing NF-κB expression [107]. Notably, salidroside has highly effective antiviral effects. Salidroside used as an adaptogen in traditional Chinese medicine and possesses a wide range of pharmacological characteristics, including anti-hypoxia, anti-aging, anti-cancer, anti-inflammatory, antioxidant, antiviral, immune-stimulating activity, anti-diabetic, etc. [109]. Nowadays, it can not only be isolated from Rhodiola species, but also be obtained through synthetic pathways [109]. Animal experiments show that salidroside exhibits antiviral activity against coxsackievirus B3 (CVB3) [106] and Influenza A virus (IAV) [108], suggesting its potential as a promising therapeutic agent for bunyavirus infections.

RNA agonists of RIG-I can enhance the IFN antiviral immune response. RNA agonists of RIG-I are widely used in preclinical and clinical studies for cancer and viral therapy. Some of the identified RNA agonists of RIG-I include 3p10LG9 [113], 5′-ppp RNA [115], 5′-ppp siRNA [111], 3p-siRNA-MDR1 [110], SLR14 [114], etc. RNA agonists of RLR can be delivered in vivo through nanoparticles, extracellular vesicles, and CAR-T cells [180]. For instance, in vitro studies demonstrated the practicality of biocompatible gold nanorod GNR-5′PPP-ssRNA, a nano-complexes as an antiviral strategy against IAV [112]. Additionally, it was indicated that a novel small dsRNA hairpin, 3p10LG9, can control DENV infection [113]. Another study suggests that 5′-ppp RNA effectively blocks herpes simplex virus 1 (HSV-1) infection in vitro and in vivo through a STING-dependent mechanism [181]. Furthermore, SLR14, a stem-loop RNA, exhibits antiviral capabilities for SARS-CoV-2 infection in a mouse model [114]. Therefore, RNA agonists of RIG-I possess broad-spectrum antiviral activity and hold potential therapeutic value in treating bunyavirus infections.

Ionizing radiation (IR) stimulates cytoplasmic RIG-I to bind with small endogenous non-coding RNAs (sncRNAs), thereby inducing IFN production. Combined therapy with RLR agonists and ionizing radiation can have a radiosensitizing effect [117]. Some studies suggested that ionizing radiation has effects against the zika virus (ZIKV), influenza virus, and poliovirus. With certain intensities of X-rays, gamma rays, or UVC light, the replication and proliferation of SARS-CoV-2 in the lungs of COVID-19 patients can be non-invasively inhibited [122]. Another study showed that the combination of UV-4B and IFN-α enhances the antiviral activity against Dengue virus [116]. Similar to the DNA-damaging effect of radiation therapy, treatment with DNA-damaging agents such as doxorubicin [120], etoposide [119], teniposide [118], and oxaliplatin [121] can induce type I IFN responses and activate dendritic cells and CD8 T cells. Hence, radiation therapy and the application of DNA-damaging agents can strengthen type I IFN-mediated antiviral effects, which potentially serve as the therapeutic strategy for bunyavirus infections.

MDA5

DNA demethylation agents can simulate viral infection by inducing dsRNA that is used in cancer immunotherapy. This viral mimicry leads to an antiviral response mediated by the cytoplasmic pattern recognition receptor MDA5, followed by MAVS activation, IRF7 nuclear translocation, and upregulation of type III IFN and ISGs [125]. Finally, it enhances the IFN response triggered by viruses and represents a potential strategy for treating bunyavirus infections. DNA methyltransferase inhibitors (DNMTis) are a type of DNA demethylation agent, including 5-azacytidine (AZA) and 5-aza-2′-deoxycytidine (DAC), which are widely used in the treatment of hematological diseases [123,124]. The new oral DNMTi ASTX727, consisting of decitabine and the cytidine deaminase (CDA) inhibitor cedazuridine, was approved by the FDA in 2020 for the treatment of high-risk MDS and CMML. CC-486, an oral formulation of Aza, received FDA approval for the treatment of AML in elderly patients who achieved first remission with intensive chemotherapy [123]. Currently, DNA methyltransferase inhibitors are successfully applied in clinical hematologic malignancies, but their potential in antiviral therapy requires further exploration and research.

4.1.2. TBK1

As described above, TBK1 is an important target in the suppression of IFN response for viruses belonging to the family Phenuiviridae of order Bunyavirales, such as DBV, GTV, and HRTV. Currently, there are numerous studies on TBK1 inhibitors in tumor therapy, but there is still a lack of research on its activators and their application in antiviral therapy. Lidocaine can promote the phosphorylation of TBK1 and IRF7, as well as the activation of JNK and downstream factors such as c-Jun through the TBK1-IRF7 and JNK-AP1 signaling pathways, and then it upregulates IFNα4 via SHP2 to have antiviral potential. Moreover, lidocaine also has potential adjunctive effects in the treatment of IAV and even SARS-CoV-2 infections [126]. Therefore, it is speculated that lidocaine has antiviral efficacy against bunyavirus through upregulation of the antiviral IFN response. Additionally, research shows that lidocaine has an anti-inflammatory effect by inhibiting the activation of NF-κB and p38 MAPK, which is a new therapeutic agent for the treatment of allergic rhinitis (AR) [182]. As a consequence, we presume that lidocaine has a potential therapeutic effect on cytokine storms triggered by bunyavirus. Further studies are required to investigate the potential of lidocaine to treat bunyavirus infections.

4.1.3. IRF3

PUUV, TULV, and SFSV can inhibit the activity of IRF3, thereby reducing the IFN induction. So, the following compounds targeting IRF3 may be applied to the treatment of bunyavirus in the future.

Isoflavone and isoflavone-like compounds are potential therapeutic agents for bunyavirus infections. Isoflavone compounds belong to the class of flavonoids and serve as specific activators of the innate immune signaling pathway, leading to the activation and nuclear translocation of IRF3, eventually demonstrating high antiviral activity against HCV and influenza virus. KIN 101, an isoflavone compound, exhibits broad-spectrum antiviral activity against DNA and RNA viruses [127]. Isoflavone and isoflavone-like compounds showed antiviral properties both in vitro and in vivo. Among them, genistein, a soy-derived isoflavone, was extensively studied for its antiviral activity and was proven to inhibit the infectivity of enveloped or non-enveloped viruses, as well as single-stranded or double-stranded RNA or DNA viruses [128].

Previous research found that the hydroxyquinoline family compounds including KIN1400 and its derivatives, KIN1408 and KIN1409, possess broad-spectrum antiviral activity. These compounds selectively activate IRF3 to promote cellular IFN response, which demonstrates their antiviral efficacy. They can prevent or treat various RNA virus infections in cell cultures, such as West Nile virus (WNV), DENV, HCV, IAV, RSV, Nipah virus (NiV), Lassa virus (LASV), and EBOV [129]. Briefly, small molecules of the hydroxyquinoline family, such as KIN1400 and its derivatives KIN1408 and KIN1409, may exhibit activity against bunyavirus by strengthening the IFN antiviral effect induced by bunyavirus.

Additionally, vaccinia virus (VACV) and bunyavirus share similarities in their ability to inhibit IFN antiviral responses. Research designed and indicated that a recombinant VACV vaccine that expresses IRF-3 in mice induces a robust protective immune response against lethal VACV in mice [183]. This finding is significant for the development of bunyavirus vaccines.

4.1.4. Others

Additionally, besides directly targeting key points in the IFN response induction and antiviral signaling as discussed above, there are several indirectly targeted therapy strategies with significant clinical value. While some of the directly targeted drugs or strategies are still in the pre-clinical research stage and require further exploration for their clinical application, some indirectly targeted drugs are widely used in clinical settings and were suggested to be closely associated with various viral infections. These indirect strategies that target IFN induction and its antiviral signaling pathway hold promise as effective measures in the treatment of bunyavirus infections. The following will discuss and summarize these potential therapeutic strategies of indirect targeting one by one.

The p97 complex promotes the proteasomal degradation of RIG-I, thereby reducing the antiviral innate immune response. Disruption of the p97 complex enhances antiviral signal transduction of RIG-I. Furthermore, P97 activity was proven to be crucial for the replication of viruses such as poliovirus, HSV, cytomegalovirus (CMV), influenza virus, etc. [130]. Currently, there are many p97 inhibitors including active sites and allosteric inhibitors. Although the drug clotrimazole was identified as a p97 inhibitor, its antiviral properties were not demonstrated [130,131]. In conclusion, it is a potential indirectly targeted therapy approach to target the p97 complex for treating bunyavirus infections. Further, p97 inhibitors along with clotrimazole may be used for the treatment of bunyavirus infections.

Mounting evidence shows that TBK1 plays an important role in the mechanism of IFN suppression in bunyavirus infections. There is a substantial amount of domestic and international research on estrogen-related receptor alpha (ERRα), especially its antitumor effects. Meanwhile, some studies indicated that ERRα can inhibit the induction of type I IFN, primarily through its interaction with TBK1 [133]. Additionally, it was suggested that ERRα is a potential target for treating human cytomegalovirus infection [134]. Therefore, targeting ERRα indirectly to modulate IFN induction by reducing ERRα activity can enhance the antiviral IFN response, which is expected to be used for controlling bunyavirus infections. It was discovered that XCT790 is a potent ERRα inverse agonist with antiviral efficacy, which is demonstrated to be effective against VSV, Newcastle disease virus (NDV), HSV, and HBV by regulating the IFN response [133,141]. Moreover, compounds such as N-[(2Z)-3-(4,5-dihydro-1,3-thiazol-2-yl)-1,3-thiazolidin-2-ylidene]-5H dibenzo[a,-d] [7]annulen-5-amine [132], kaempferol [137], cyclohexylmethyl-(1-p-tolyl-1H-indol-3-ylmethyl)-amine [135], LingH2-10 [139], naringenin [138], and SR16388 [140] were all identified to inhibit ERRα activity. Furthermore, research identified five anticancer drugs and nine pesticides capable of inhibiting ERRα activity [136]. Briefly, numerous drugs and compounds were identified as potential ERRα inhibitors with promising prospects for the treatment of bunyavirus infections that hold significant research value.

Just as mentioned above, IRF3 is a critical target for the mechanisms of IFN suppression in bunyavirus infections. The deficiency of 7-dehydrocholesterol reductase (DHCR7) or treatment with natural product 7-dehydrocholesterol (7-DHC) can specifically promote the phosphorylation of IRF3, thereby enhancing the production of type I IFN in macrophages [149]. Notably, DHCR7 deficiency and DHCR7 inhibitors such as AY9944 and the chemotherapeutic drug Tamoxifen promote the clearance of various viruses both in vitro and in vivo. It was shown that they can inhibit ZIKV, vesicular stomatitis virus (VSV), HCV, HSV, and SARS-CoV-2 infections [146–149]. Therefore, DHCR7 inhibitors and 7-DHC can enhance the innate antiviral immune response triggered by viral infections and may be used in the treatment of bunyavirus infections. There were some DHCR7 inhibitors identified among existing drugs, including Tamoxifen [142] and antipsychotic drugs such as haloperidol, aripiprazole, cariprazine, and trazodone [143,144]. Likewise, small molecules such as AY9944 and BM15.766 were confirmed to effectively inhibit DHCR7 [145,150]. Overall, these DHCR7 inhibitors hold potential as drugs for treating bunyavirus infections by indirectly targeting IRF3.

The bunyaviruses SNV and SFSV inhibit IFN signaling by interfering with the JAK-STAT pathway. In the JAK-STAT pathway, there is a suppressor of cytokine signaling called SOCS. SOCS-1 and SOCS-3 are the main members of the SOCS protein family, but they act differently. SOCS-1 directly binds to the JAK kinase domain to inhibit phosphorylation, while SOCS-3 binds directly to JAK kinases and cytokine receptors to inhibit JAK-STAT signaling [184]. SOCS1 and SOCS3 are intrinsic virulence factors for some virus infections, such as influenza A virus, encephalomyocarditis virus, HSV-1, vaccinia virus (VV), DENV, Zika virus, WNV, and EBOV [154]. Taken together, SOCS antagonists can serve as a method for treating these viral infections. Furthermore, research developed a small peptide antagonist of SOCS-1 called pJAK2 (1001–1013), which can prevent HSV-1 [152], IAV, VV [153], and encephalomyocarditis virus (EMCV) infections and inhibit their replication, demonstrating broad antiviral activity [151]. Consequently, it is feasible to target SOCS proteins indirectly to regulate JAK-STAT signaling in diseases. SOCS antagonists can enhance JAK-STAT signaling and then strengthen the IFN response to achieve antiviral effects. SOCS proteins represent potential targets for the treatment of bunyavirus infections, and SOCS antagonists such as pJAK2 (1001–1013) are potential compounds for treating bunyavirus infections.

MEK regulates the type I IFN response of human primary airway epithelial cells. There is evidence that MEK inhibitors (MEKi) can strengthen the type I IFN response after infecting with respiratory viruses rhinovirus (RV2) or respiratory syncytial virus (RSVA2) mainly by promoting the expression of IFN-β and the translation of ISGs [156]. In addition, trametinib was approved as a MEKi that inhibits the induction of IFN-β and then effectively blocks the replication of various subtypes of influenza A viruses in vitro and in vivo [155,157]. Therefore, trametinib, the MEKi, is expected to be used for bunyavirus infections by enhancing the type I IFN response.

4.2. *Targeting Viral Proteins*

4.2.1. NSs

NSs are essential for many bunyaviruses (BUNV, LACV, DBV, RVFV, SFSV, etc.) to inhibit IFN response and mediate immune evasion. While there is currently a lack of research on therapeutic strategies targeting bunyavirus NSs, numerous studies demonstrated the potential value of using DENV NS1 as a therapeutic target and candidate vaccine. The approaches and methods of these studies hold significant insights and references for exploring antiviral treatment strategies targeting bunyavirus NSs. A study investigated the drug-like properties, binding affinity, interaction of plant compounds and DENV NS1 protein, and the interaction of NS1 and TLR4 through pharmacokinetics, molecular docking, binding affinity, interaction, and molecular dynamics. They found that three plant compounds named rutin, myricetin 3-rhamnoside, and kaempferol 3-(2″-rhamnosylrutinoside) bind to the critical amino acid residue ASN130 at the active site of the NS1 protein, thus improving platelet reduction in DENV-infected patients by disrupting the interaction of NS1 and TLR4 [185]. Another molecular docking-based study discovered that plant flavonoids can also bind to the ASN130 glycosylation site of DENV NS1 to potentially inhibit virus replication. These flavonoids are hopeful to be antiviral drugs for DENV infection [186]. Furthermore, there is evidence that anti-NS1 antibodies can serve as specific therapeutic drugs for dengue virus infection to block NS1-induced pathogenic effects both in vitro and in vivo, which reduce virus replication and lower mortality and morbidity in different mouse models of DENV infection [187,188]. NS1 is a candidate vaccine for DENV infection, as it can trigger both cellular and humoral immunity. Studies indicated that the mice inoculated with DENV NS1 by different methods can possess protective immune responses against DENV infection [189–191].

RNA interference (RNAi) is a method used to silence viral genes, and small interfering RNA (siRNA) was demonstrated as a potential therapeutic strategy against viral infections [161]. The siRNA that specifically targets the non-structural protein genes for various viruses such as IAV [158], porcine reproductive and respiratory syndrome virus (PRRSV) [160], WNV [159], and SARS-CoV-2 [162] can reduce viral titers, thereby inhibiting viral infections. In terms of bunyaviruses, there is a study indicating that RNAi activators have potential therapeutic benefits against RVFV infections. In a cell culture model of RVFV replication, short hairpin RNAs (shRNA) targeting the N gene reduced intracellular nucleocapsid protein concentration and viral replication, while shRNA targeting the NSs gene reduced NSs protein concentration, thereby alleviating NS-mediated cytotoxicity [192]. However, there is evidence that LACV, a member of the California serogroup of orthobunyaviruses, may have the capability to inhibit RNAi [193,194]. Therefore, RNAi-based viral gene silencing may be ineffective against LACV infection. In summary, siRNA targeting the NS gene of bunyaviruses can reduce NS expression, thereby inhibiting its antagonistic effect on IFN, which can provide antiviral benefits in bunyaviruses excluding LACV infection.

4.2.2. NP

In the interference mechanism of IFN suppression in HTNV, NP plays a crucial role. NP can inhibit the NF-κB activity in the IFN antiviral pathway through various pathways. Therefore, targeting HTNV's NP can counteract the virus's immune escape mechanisms, presenting a potential strategy for treating HTNV infections. Various antiviral treatment approaches targeting the viral NP were extensively explored.

For instance, Sharifi et al. employed virtual screening through docking followed by molecular dynamics and discovered that doxycycline and minocycline are potential inhibitors of CCHFV NP [163]. Additionally, IAV's NP is a critical target for antiviral therapy. Compounds such as curcumin [166] and naproxen [168] inhibit the NP-RNA binding required for IAV NP function, serving as novel antiviral drugs against IAV. Curcumin derivatives, such as tetramethylcurcumin, also exhibit inhibitory effects against IAV [195]. Furthermore, curcumin and its derivatives control EBOV infection by targeting NP [164] and demonstrate broad-spectrum antiviral activity against HIV, DENV, HSV-2, and other viruses [165]. Similarly, naproxen was found to target the NP of SARS-CoV-2, exhibiting antiviral properties [167]. Therefore, curcumin and naproxen, especially curcumin, may be potential candidates for HTNV treatment, warranting further research for validation. Compound RK424 [169] demonstrated effective antiviral activity against IAV by inhibiting NP's RNA binding, oligomerization, and nuclear export functions, and validated in vitro and mouse models.

RNAi targeting the NS gene and RNAi targeting the NP gene through siRNA and shRNA provide a direct and rapid treatment for viral infections, proving to be effective against various viruses such as human metapneumovirus (hMPV) [171], rabies virus [170], Borna disease virus (BoDV-1) [173], and IAV [172]], which is a potential measure to treat HTNV infection. Moreover, NP-specific monoclonal antibodies (mAbs) were extensively developed for antiviral therapy against IAV [174]. Antisense oligonucleotides designed for the NP gene's RNA binding region inhibit the replication of highly pathogenic avian influenza virus (AIV) H5N1, representing a novel therapeutic candidate [175]. These approaches offer new avenues for the treatment of HTNV infections.

4.2.3. GPC

GPC participates in IFN suppression in PUUV and SNV and is a potential target for antiviral therapy. Research indicates that some antiviral treatments act by targeting GPC. Trametinib, for example, inhibits GPC-mediated membrane fusion by targeting the transmembrane (TM) domain of Lujo virus (LUJV) GPC, making it a candidate drug for treating LUJV infections [176]. Additionally, it was mentioned above that trametinib, as a MEK inhibitor, is also expected to be used for bunyavirus infections. Therefore, trametinib holds significant research value for the treatment of PUUV and SNV. Additionally, the proprotein-processing protease furin inhibitor, decanoyl-Arg-Val-Lys-Arg-chloromethylketone (dec-RVKR-cmk), exhibits antiviral activity [196] and is a potential drug for treating SARS-CoV-2 and HBV [197]. Furthermore, research indicates that decanoyl-RRLL-chloromethylketone (dec-RRLL-cmk), the inhibitors of the cellular proprotein convertase site 1 protease (S1P), targeting GPC, can specifically block the transmission and generation of lymphocytic choriomeningitis virus (LCMV) [198]. Developing drugs as inhibitors of GPC's processing protease holds promise for treating PUUV or SNV infections.

4.2.4. Gn

Gn and Gc play a role in IFN suppression mechanisms in HTNV and PUUV, which are potential targets for antiviral therapy. However, there is currently a lack of reported treatment strategies specifically targeting the viral Gn or Gc. Research suggests that 2-

deoxy-D-glucose (2-DG), the glycolysis inhibitor, inhibits LCMV propagation by targeting glycoprotein N-glycosylation [177]. Additionally, the Drug Controller General of India gave emergency approval for 2-DG in COVID-19 patients, and 2-DG exhibits antiviral activity against HPV18, rhinoviruses (RV), HBV, HSV, etc [178]. Therefore, 2-DG is a promising drug for treating HTNV or PUUV infections, requiring further exploration and validation.

5. Conclusions

Some species of the order Bunyavirales exert a significant impact on public health. IFN response suppression is a crucial mechanism for immune evasion following the invasion of the host by bunyaviruses which is a critical determining factor in the pathogenicity. Within this viral order, the targets involved in IFN inhibition exhibit similarities while also presenting certain differences. A large number of potential therapeutic approaches against the IFN response suppression of bunyavirus are presented in this article, which provide references for both the following basic research and practical applications. The research on drugs or compounds targeting the IFN response pathway may potentially offer novel choices and perspectives for antiviral treatments. According to their drug development, antiviral research, and clinical application, we conclude that trametinib, tamoxifen, nitazoxanide, acitretin, salidroside, curcumin, genistein, MSCs, radiotherapy, and DNA damage agents have great clinical application prospects in the treatment of bunyavirus infection.

Author Contributions: Conceptualization, Z.Z. and J.Z.; writing—original draft preparation, Y.H., M.S., X.W., A.Y. and B.L.; writing—review and editing, Z.Z. and J.Z.; supervision, Z.Z.; project administration, J.Z. and Y.H.; funding acquisition, Z.Z. All authors have read and agreed to the published version of the manuscript.

Funding: The study was supported by the Anhui Provincial Natural Science Foundation [Grant number: 2108085MH298]. The funders had no role in the study design, data collection, analysis, decision to publish, or manuscript preparation.

Conflicts of Interest: The authors declare no conflict of interest.

References

1. Boshra, H. An Overview of the Infectious Cycle of Bunyaviruses. *Viruses* **2022**, *14*, 2139. [CrossRef] [PubMed]
2. Elliott, R.M.; Weber, F. Bunyaviruses and the type I interferon system. *Viruses* **2009**, *1*, 1003–1021. [CrossRef]
3. Spengler, J.R.; Bente, D.A.; Bray, M.; Burt, F.; Hewson, R.; Korukluoglu, G.; Mirazimi, A.; Weber, F.; Papa, A. Second International Conference on Crimean-Congo Hemorrhagic Fever. *Antivir. Res.* **2018**, *150*, 137–147. [CrossRef] [PubMed]
4. Matthews, E.; Chauhan, L.; Piquet, A.L.; Tyler, K.L.; Pastula, D.M. An Overview of La Crosse Virus Disease. *Neurohospitalist* **2022**, *12*, 587–588. [CrossRef] [PubMed]
5. Overturf, G.D. World arboviruses: The Bunyaviridae. *Pediatr. Infect. Dis. J.* **2009**, *28*, 1014–1015. [CrossRef] [PubMed]
6. Anderson, G.W.; Slayter, M.V.; Hall, W.; Peters, C.J. Pathogenesis of a phleboviral infection (Punta Toro virus) in golden Syrian hamsters. *Arch. Virol.* **1990**, *114*, 203–212. [CrossRef]
7. Perrone, L.A.; Narayanan, K.; Worthy, M.; Peters, C.J. The S segment of Punta Toro virus (Bunyaviridae, Phlebovirus) is a major determinant of lethality in the Syrian hamster and codes for a type I interferon antagonist. *J. Virol.* **2007**, *81*, 884–892. [CrossRef]
8. Isaacs, A.; Lindenmann, J. Virus interference. I. The interferon. *Proc. R. Soc. Lond. B Biol. Sci.* **1957**, *147*, 258–267.
9. Barnas, J.L.; Albrecht, J.; Meednu, N.; Alzamareh, D.F.; Baker, C.; McDavid, A.; Looney, R.J.; Anolik, J.H. B Cell Activation and Plasma Cell Differentiation Are Promoted by IFN-λ in Systemic Lupus Erythematosus. *J. Immunol.* **2021**, *207*, 2660–2672. [CrossRef]
10. Vazquez, M.I.; Catalan-Dibene, J.; Zlotnik, A. B cells responses and cytokine production are regulated by their immune microenvironment. *Cytokine* **2015**, *74*, 318–326. [CrossRef]
11. Fink, K.; Lang, K.S.; Manjarrez-Orduno, N.; Junt, T.; Senn, B.M.; Holdener, M.; Akira, S.; Zinkernagel, R.M.; Hengartner, H. Early type I interferon-mediated signals on B cells specifically enhance antiviral humoral responses. *Eur. J. Immunol.* **2006**, *36*, 2094–2105. [CrossRef]
12. Giordani, L.; Sanchez, M.; Libri, I.; Quaranta, M.G.; Mattioli, B.; Viora, M. IFN-α amplifies human naive B cell TLR-9-mediated activation and Ig production. *J. Leukoc. Biol.* **2009**, *86*, 261–271. [CrossRef]
13. Samuel, C.E. Antiviral actions of interferons. *Clin. Microbiol. Rev.* **2001**, *14*, 778–809. [CrossRef]

14. Hamana, A.; Takahashi, Y.; Uchida, T.; Nishikawa, M.; Imamura, M.; Chayama, K.; Takakura, Y. Evaluation of antiviral effect of type I, II, and III interferons on direct-acting antiviral-resistant hepatitis C virus. *Antivir. Res.* **2017**, *146*, 130–138. [CrossRef] [PubMed]
15. Zhang, Z.; Ni, Y.; Lempp, F.A.; Walter, L.; Mutz, P.; Bartenschlager, R.; Urban, S. Hepatitis D virus-induced interferon response and administered interferons control cell division-mediated virus spread. *J. Hepatol.* **2022**, *77*, 957–966. [CrossRef]
16. Yin, Y.; Favoreel, H.W. Herpesviruses and the Type III Interferon System. *Virol. Sin.* **2021**, *36*, 577–587. [CrossRef] [PubMed]
17. Ank, N.; West, H.; Paludan, S.R. IFN-lambda: Novel antiviral cytokines. *J. Interferon Cytokine Res.* **2006**, *26*, 373–379. [CrossRef] [PubMed]
18. Aricò, E.; Belardelli, F. Interferon-α as antiviral and antitumor vaccine adjuvants: Mechanisms of action and response signature. *J. Interferon Cytokine Res.* **2012**, *32*, 235–247. [CrossRef] [PubMed]
19. Zhou, H.; Chen, S.; Wang, M.; Cheng, A. Interferons and their receptors in birds: A comparison of gene structure, phylogenetic analysis, and cross modulation. *Int. J. Mol. Sci.* **2014**, *15*, 21045–21068. [CrossRef]
20. Kotenko, S.V. IFN-λs. *Curr. Opin. Immunol.* **2011**, *23*, 583–590. [CrossRef]
21. Lazear, H.M.; Schoggins, J.W.; Diamond, M.S. Shared and Distinct Functions of Type I and Type III Interferons. *Immunity* **2019**, *50*, 907–923. [CrossRef] [PubMed]
22. Dowling, J.W.; Forero, A. Beyond Good and Evil: Molecular Mechanisms of Type I and III IFN Functions. *J. Immunol.* **2022**, *208*, 247–256. [CrossRef]
23. Nallar, S.C.; Kalvakolanu, D.V. Interferons, signal transduction pathways, and the central nervous system. *J. Interferon Cytokine Res.* **2014**, *34*, 559–576. [CrossRef] [PubMed]
24. Durbin, R.K.; Kotenko, S.V.; Durbin, J.E. Interferon induction and function at the mucosal surface. *Immunol. Rev.* **2013**, *255*, 25–39. [CrossRef]
25. Ioannidis, I.; McNally, B.; Willette, M.; Peeples, M.E.; Chaussabel, D.; Durbin, J.E.; Ramilo, O.; Mejias, A.; Flaño, E. Plasticity and virus specificity of the airway epithelial cell immune response during respiratory virus infection. *J. Virol.* **2012**, *86*, 5422–5436. [CrossRef] [PubMed]
26. Kawai, T.; Akira, S. Toll-like receptors and their crosstalk with other innate receptors in infection and immunity. *Immunity* **2011**, *34*, 637–650. [CrossRef] [PubMed]
27. Takeda, K.; Akira, S. Toll-like receptors in innate immunity. *Int. Immunol.* **2005**, *17*, 1–14. [CrossRef]
28. Li, Y.; Chen, R.; Zhou, Q.; Xu, Z.; Li, C.; Wang, S.; Mao, A.; Zhang, X.; He, W.; Shu, H.-B. LSm14A is a processing body-associated sensor of viral nucleic acids that initiates cellular antiviral response in the early phase of viral infection. *Proc. Natl. Acad. Sci. USA* **2012**, *109*, 11770–11775. [CrossRef]
29. Rahimi-Tesiye, M.; Zaersabet, M.; Salehiyeh, S.; Jafari, S.Z. The role of TRIM25 in the occurrence and development of cancers and inflammatory diseases. *Biochim. Biophys. Acta Rev. Cancer* **2023**, *1878*, 188954. [CrossRef]
30. Kawai, T.; Akira, S. The roles of TLRs, RLRs and NLRs in pathogen recognition. *Int. Immunol.* **2009**, *21*, 317–337. [CrossRef]
31. Radetskyy, R.; Daher, A.; Gatignol, A. ADAR1 and PKR, interferon stimulated genes with clashing effects on HIV-1 replication. *Cytokine Growth Factor Rev.* **2018**, *40*, 48–58. [CrossRef]
32. Weiss, C.M.; Trobaugh, D.W.; Sun, C.; Lucas, T.M.; Diamond, M.S.; Ryman, K.D.; Klimstra, W.B. The Interferon-Induced Exonuclease ISG20 Exerts Antiviral Activity through Upregulation of Type I Interferon Response Proteins. *mSphere* **2018**, *3*, e00209-18. [CrossRef] [PubMed]
33. Mirzalieva, O.; Juncker, M.; Schwartzenburg, J.; Desai, S. ISG15 and ISGylation in Human Diseases. *Cells* **2022**, *11*, 538. [CrossRef] [PubMed]
34. Content, J. Mechanisms of induction and action of interferons. *Verh. K. Acad. Geneeskd. Belg.* **2009**, *71*, 51–71. [PubMed]
35. de Weerd, N.A.; Samarajiwa, S.A.; Hertzog, P.J. Type I interferon receptors: Biochemistry and biological functions. *J. Biol. Chem.* **2007**, *282*, 20053–20057. [CrossRef]
36. Müller, M.; Briscoe, J.; Laxton, C.; Guschin, D.; Ziemiecki, A.; Silvennoinen, O.; Harpur, A.G.; Barbieri, G.; Witthuhn, B.A.; Schindler, C. The protein tyrosine kinase JAK1 complements defects in interferon-α/β and -γ signal transduction. *Nature* **1993**, *366*, 129–135. [CrossRef]
37. Greenlund, A.C.; Morales, M.O.; Viviano, B.L.; Yan, H.; Krolewski, J.; Schreiber, R.D. Stat recruitment by tyrosine-phosphorylated cytokine receptors: An ordered reversible affinity-driven process. *Immunity* **1995**, *2*, 677–687. [CrossRef]
38. Randall, R.E.; Goodbourn, S. Interferons and viruses: An interplay between induction, signalling, antiviral responses and virus countermeasures. *J. Gen. Virol.* **2008**, *89*, 1–47. [CrossRef]
39. Negishi, H.; Taniguchi, T.; Yanai, H. The Interferon (IFN) Class of Cytokines and the IFN Regulatory Factor (IRF) Transcription Factor Family. *Cold Spring Harb. Perspect. Biol.* **2018**, *10*, a028423. [CrossRef]
40. Odendall, C.; Dixit, E.; Stavru, F.; Bierne, H.; Franz, K.M.; Durbin, A.F.; Boulant, S.; Gehrke, L.; Cossart, P.; Kagan, J.C. Diverse intracellular pathogens activate type III interferon expression from peroxisomes. *Nat. Immunol.* **2014**, *15*, 717–726. [CrossRef]
41. Zhou, Z.; Hamming, O.J.; Ank, N.; Paludan, S.R.; Nielsen, A.L.; Hartmann, R. Type III interferon (IFN) induces a type I IFN-like response in a restricted subset of cells through signaling pathways involving both the Jak-STAT pathway and the mitogen-activated protein kinases. *J. Virol.* **2007**, *81*, 7749–7758. [CrossRef] [PubMed]

42. Kotenko, S.V.; Gallagher, G.; Baurin, V.V.; Lewis-Antes, A.; Shen, M.; Shah, N.K.; Langer, J.A.; Sheikh, F.; Dickensheets, H.; Donnelly, R.P. IFN-lambdas mediate antiviral protection through a distinct class II cytokine receptor complex. *Nat. Immunol.* **2003**, *4*, 69–77. [CrossRef] [PubMed]
43. Thuner, J.; Coutant, F. IFN-γ: An overlooked cytokine in dermatomyositis with anti-MDA5 antibodies. *Autoimmun. Rev.* **2023**, *22*, 103420. [CrossRef] [PubMed]
44. Schroder, K.; Hertzog, P.J.; Ravasi, T.; Hume, D.A. Interferon-gamma: An overview of signals, mechanisms and functions. *J. Leukoc. Biol.* **2004**, *75*, 163–189. [CrossRef] [PubMed]
45. Kak, G.; Raza, M.; Tiwari, B.K. Interferon-gamma (IFN-γ): Exploring its implications in infectious diseases. *Biomol. Concepts* **2018**, *9*, 64–79. [CrossRef]
46. Biron, C.A.; Nguyen, K.B.; Pien, G.C.; Cousens, L.P.; Salazar-Mather, T.P. Natural killer cells in antiviral defense: Function and regulation by innate cytokines. *Annu. Rev. Immunol.* **1999**, *17*, 189–220. [CrossRef]
47. Fenimore, J.; Young, H.A. Regulation of IFN-γ Expression. *Adv. Exp. Med. Biol.* **2016**, *941*, 1–19.
48. Zundler, S.; Neurath, M.F. Interleukin-12: Functional activities and implications for disease. *Cytokine Growth Factor Rev.* **2015**, *26*, 559–568. [CrossRef]
49. Santiago, F.W.; Covaleda, L.M.; Sanchez-Aparicio, M.T.; Silvas, J.A.; Diaz-Vizarreta, A.C.; Patel, J.R.; Popov, V.; Yu, X.-j.; García-Sastre, A.; Aguilar, P.V. Hijacking of RIG-I signaling proteins into virus-induced cytoplasmic structures correlates with the inhibition of type I interferon responses. *J. Virol.* **2014**, *88*, 4572–4585. [CrossRef]
50. Min, Y.-Q.; Ning, Y.-J.; Wang, H.; Deng, F. A RIG-I-like receptor directs antiviral responses to a bunyavirus and is antagonized by virus-induced blockade of TRIM25-mediated ubiquitination. *J. Biol. Chem.* **2020**, *295*, 9691–9711. [CrossRef]
51. Zhang, S.; Zheng, B.; Wang, T.; Li, A.; Wan, J.; Qu, J.; Li, C.H.; Li, D.; Liang, M. NSs protein of severe fever with thrombocytopenia syndrome virus suppresses interferon production through different mechanism than Rift Valley fever virus. *Acta Virol.* **2017**, *61*, 289–298. [CrossRef] [PubMed]
52. Moriyama, M.; Igarashi, M.; Koshiba, T.; Irie, T.; Takada, A.; Ichinohe, T. Two Conserved Amino Acids within the NSs of Severe Fever with Thrombocytopenia Syndrome Phlebovirus Are Essential for Anti-Interferon Activity. *J. Virol.* **2018**, *92*, e00706–e00718. [CrossRef] [PubMed]
53. Kitagawa, Y.; Sakai, M.; Shimojima, M.; Saijo, M.; Itoh, M.; Gotoh, B. Nonstructural protein of severe fever with thrombocytopenia syndrome phlebovirus targets STAT2 and not STAT1 to inhibit type I interferon-stimulated JAK-STAT signaling. *Microbes Infect.* **2018**, *20*, 360–368. [CrossRef] [PubMed]
54. Hong, Y.; Bai, M.; Qi, X.; Li, C.; Liang, M.; Li, D.; Cardona, C.J.; Xing, Z. Suppression of the IFN-α and -β Induction through Sequestering IRF7 into Viral Inclusion Bodies by Nonstructural Protein NSs in Severe Fever with Thrombocytopenia Syndrome Bunyavirus Infection. *J. Immunol.* **2019**, *202*, 841–856. [CrossRef]
55. Ning, Y.-J.; Feng, K.; Min, Y.-Q.; Cao, W.-C.; Wang, M.; Deng, F.; Hu, Z.; Wang, H. Disruption of type I interferon signaling by the nonstructural protein of severe fever with thrombocytopenia syndrome virus via the hijacking of STAT2 and STAT1 into inclusion bodies. *J. Virol.* **2015**, *89*, 4227–4236. [CrossRef]
56. Zhang, L.; Fu, Y.; Zhang, R.; Guan, Y.; Jiang, N.; Zheng, N.; Wu, Z. Nonstructural Protein NSs Hampers Cellular Antiviral Response through LSm14A during Severe Fever with Thrombocytopenia Syndrome Virus Infection. *J. Immunol.* **2021**, *207*, 590–601. [CrossRef]
57. Min, Y.-Q.; Shi, C.; Yao, T.; Feng, K.; Mo, Q.; Deng, F.; Wang, H.; Ning, Y.-J. The Nonstructural Protein of Guertu Virus Disrupts Host Defenses by Blocking Antiviral Interferon Induction and Action. *ACS Infect. Dis.* **2020**, *6*, 857–870. [CrossRef]
58. Feng, K.; Deng, F.; Hu, Z.; Wang, H.; Ning, Y.-J. Heartland virus antagonizes type I and III interferon antiviral signaling by inhibiting phosphorylation and nuclear translocation of STAT2 and STAT1. *J. Biol. Chem.* **2019**, *294*, 9503–9517. [CrossRef]
59. Ning, Y.-J.; Feng, K.; Min, Y.-Q.; Deng, F.; Hu, Z.; Wang, H. Heartland virus NSs protein disrupts host defenses by blocking the TBK1 kinase-IRF3 transcription factor interaction and signaling required for interferon induction. *J. Biol. Chem.* **2017**, *292*, 16722–16733. [CrossRef]
60. Holzer, B.; Bakshi, S.; Bridgen, A.; Baron, M.D. Inhibition of interferon induction and action by the nairovirus Nairobi sheep disease virus/Ganjam virus. *PLoS ONE* **2011**, *6*, e28594. [CrossRef]
61. Ermler, M.E.; Yerukhim, E.; Schriewer, J.; Schattgen, S.; Traylor, Z.; Wespiser, A.R.; Caffrey, D.R.; Chen, Z.J.; King, C.H.; Gale, M.; et al. RNA helicase signaling is critical for type I interferon production and protection against Rift Valley fever virus during mucosal challenge. *J. Virol.* **2013**, *87*, 4846–4860. [CrossRef] [PubMed]
62. Billecocq, A.; Spiegel, M.; Vialat, P.; Kohl, A.; Weber, F.; Bouloy, M.; Haller, O. NSs protein of Rift Valley fever virus blocks interferon production by inhibiting host gene transcription. *J. Virol.* **2004**, *78*, 9798–9806. [CrossRef] [PubMed]
63. Habjan, M.; Pichlmair, A.; Elliott, R.M.; Overby, A.K.; Glatter, T.; Gstaiger, M.; Superti-Furga, G.; Unger, H.; Weber, F. NSs protein of rift valley fever virus induces the specific degradation of the double-stranded RNA-dependent protein kinase. *J. Virol.* **2009**, *83*, 4365–4375. [CrossRef]
64. Gowen, B.B.; Bailey, K.W.; Scharton, D.; Vest, Z.; Westover, J.B.; Skirpstunas, R.; Ikegami, T. Post-exposure vaccination with MP-12 lacking NSs protects mice against lethal Rift Valley fever virus challenge. *Antivir. Res.* **2013**, *98*, 135–143. [CrossRef] [PubMed]
65. Le May, N.; Mansuroglu, Z.; Léger, P.; Josse, T.; Blot, G.; Billecocq, A.; Flick, R.; Jacob, Y.; Bonnefoy, E.; Bouloy, M. A SAP30 complex inhibits IFN-β expression in Rift Valley fever virus infected cells. *PLoS Pathog.* **2008**, *4*, e13. [CrossRef]

66. Ikegami, T.; Narayanan, K.; Won, S.; Kamitani, W.; Peters, C.J.; Makino, S. Rift Valley fever virus NSs protein promotes post-transcriptional downregulation of protein kinase PKR and inhibits eIF2α phosphorylation. *PLoS Pathog.* **2009**, *5*, e1000287. [CrossRef]
67. Feng, J.; De Jesus, P.D.; Su, V.; Han, S.; Gong, D.; Wu, N.C.; Tian, Y.; Li, X.; Wu, T.-T.; Chanda, S.K.; et al. RIOK3 is an adaptor protein required for IRF3-mediated antiviral type I interferon production. *J. Virol.* **2014**, *88*, 7987–7997. [CrossRef]
68. Takashima, K.; Oshiumi, H.; Takaki, H.; Matsumoto, M.; Seya, T. RIOK3-mediated phosphorylation of MDA5 interferes with its assembly and attenuates the innate immune response. *Cell Rep.* **2015**, *11*, 192–200. [CrossRef]
69. Havranek, K.E.; White, L.A.; Bisom, T.C.; Lanchy, J.-M.; Lodmell, J.S. The Atypical Kinase RIOK3 Limits RVFV Propagation and Is Regulated by Alternative Splicing. *Viruses* **2021**, *13*, 367. [CrossRef]
70. Barski, M.; Brennan, B.; Miller, O.K.; Potter, J.A.; Vijayakrishnan, S.; Bhella, D.; Naismith, J.H.; Elliott, R.M.; Schwarz-Linek, U. Rift Valley fever phlebovirus NSs protein core domain structure suggests molecular basis for nuclear filaments. *eLife* **2017**, *6*, e29236. [CrossRef]
71. Wuerth, J.D.; Habjan, M.; Wulle, J.; Superti-Furga, G.; Pichlmair, A.; Weber, F. NSs Protein of Sandfly Fever Sicilian Phlebovirus Counteracts Interferon (IFN) Induction by Masking the DNA-Binding Domain of IFN Regulatory Factor 3. *J. Virol.* **2018**, *92*, e01202–e01218. [CrossRef]
72. Moalem, Y.; Malis, Y.; Voloshin, K.; Dukhovny, A.; Hirschberg, K.; Sklan, E.H. Sandfly Fever Viruses Attenuate the Type I Interferon Response by Targeting the Phosphorylation of JAK-STAT Components. *Front. Immunol.* **2022**, *13*, 865797. [CrossRef]
73. Ito, T.; Wuerth, J.D.; Weber, F. Protection of eIF2B from inhibitory phosphorylated eIF2: A viral strategy to maintain mRNA translation during the PKR-triggered integrated stress response. *J. Biol. Chem.* **2023**, *299*, 105287. [CrossRef] [PubMed]
74. Taylor, S.L.; Frias-Staheli, N.; García-Sastre, A.; Schmaljohn, C.S. Hantaan virus nucleocapsid protein binds to importin alpha proteins and inhibits tumor necrosis factor alpha-induced activation of nuclear factor kappa B. *J. Virol.* **2009**, *83*, 1271–1279. [CrossRef] [PubMed]
75. Taylor, S.L.; Krempel, R.L.; Schmaljohn, C.S. Inhibition of TNF-α-induced activation of NF-κB by hantavirus nucleocapsid proteins. *Ann. N. Y. Acad. Sci.* **2009**, *1171* (Suppl. S1), E86–E93. [CrossRef] [PubMed]
76. Pan, W.; Bian, G.; Wang, K.; Feng, T.; Dai, J. Effects of Different Doses of Nucleocapsid Protein from Hantaan Virus A9 Strain on Regulation of Interferon Signaling. *Viral Immunol.* **2015**, *28*, 448–454. [CrossRef]
77. Wang, K.; Ma, H.; Liu, H.; Ye, W.; Li, Z.; Cheng, L.; Zhang, L.; Lei, Y.; Shen, L.; Zhang, F. The Glycoprotein and Nucleocapsid Protein of Hantaviruses Manipulate Autophagy Flux to Restrain Host Innate Immune Responses. *Cell Rep.* **2019**, *27*, 2075–2091. [CrossRef]
78. Gallo, G.; Caignard, G.; Badonnel, K.; Chevreux, G.; Terrier, S.; Szemiel, A.; Roman-Sosa, G.; Binder, F.; Gu, Q.; Da Silva Filipe, A.; et al. Interactions of Viral Proteins from Pathogenic and Low or Non-Pathogenic Orthohantaviruses with Human Type I Interferon Signaling. *Viruses* **2021**, *13*, 140. [CrossRef]
79. Levine, J.R.; Prescott, J.; Brown, K.S.; Best, S.M.; Ebihara, H.; Feldmann, H. Antagonism of type I interferon responses by new world hantaviruses. *J. Virol.* **2010**, *84*, 11790–11801. [CrossRef]
80. Jääskeläinen, K.M.; Kaukinen, P.; Minskaya, E.S.; Plyusnina, A.; Vapalahti, O.; Elliott, R.M.; Weber, F.; Vaheri, A.; Plyusnin, A. Tula and Puumala hantavirus NSs ORFs are functional and the products inhibit activation of the interferon-beta promoter. *J. Med. Virol.* **2007**, *79*, 1527–1536. [CrossRef]
81. Streitenfeld, H.; Boyd, A.; Fazakerley, J.K.; Bridgen, A.; Elliott, R.M.; Weber, F. Activation of PKR by Bunyamwera virus is independent of the viral interferon antagonist NSs. *J. Virol.* **2003**, *77*, 5507–5511. [CrossRef]
82. Thomas, D.; Blakqori, G.; Wagner, V.; Banholzer, M.; Kessler, N.; Elliott, R.M.; Haller, O.; Weber, F. Inhibition of RNA polymerase II phosphorylation by a viral interferon antagonist. *J. Biol. Chem.* **2004**, *279*, 31471–31477. [CrossRef] [PubMed]
83. Carlton-Smith, C.; Elliott, R.M. Viperin, MTAP44, and protein kinase R contribute to the interferon-induced inhibition of Bunyamwera Orthobunyavirus replication. *J. Virol.* **2012**, *86*, 11548–11557. [CrossRef] [PubMed]
84. Verbruggen, P.; Ruf, M.; Blakqori, G.; Överby, A.K.; Heidemann, M.; Eick, D.; Weber, F. Interferon antagonist NSs of La Crosse virus triggers a DNA damage response-like degradation of transcribing RNA polymerase II. *J. Biol. Chem.* **2011**, *286*, 3681–3692. [CrossRef] [PubMed]
85. Schoen, A.; Lau, S.; Verbruggen, P.; Weber, F. Elongin C Contributes to RNA Polymerase II Degradation by the Interferon Antagonist NSs of La Crosse Orthobunyavirus. *J. Virol.* **2020**, *94*, e02134-19. [CrossRef]
86. de Melo Junior, A.B.; de Souza, W.M.; Acrani, G.O.; Carvalho, V.L.; Romeiro, M.F.; Tolardo, A.L.; da Silva, S.P.; Cardoso, J.F.; Chiang, J.d.O.; da Silva Goncalves Vianez Junior, J.L.; et al. Genomic characterization and evolution of Tacaiuma *orthobunyavirus* (*Peribunyaviridae* family) isolated in Brazil. *Infect. Genet. Evol.* **2018**, *60*, 71–76. [CrossRef]
87. Feng, J.; Wickenhagen, A.; Turnbull, M.L.; Rezelj, V.V.; Kreher, F.; Tilston-Lunel, N.L.; Slack, G.S.; Brennan, B.; Koudriakova, E.; Shaw, A.E.; et al. Interferon-Stimulated Gene (ISG)-Expression Screening Reveals the Specific Antibunyaviral Activity of ISG20. *J. Virol.* **2018**, *92*, e02140-17. [CrossRef]
88. Deaton, M.K.; Dzimianski, J.V.; Daczkowski, C.M.; Whitney, G.K.; Mank, N.J.; Parham, M.M.; Bergeron, E.; Pegan, S.D. Biochemical and Structural Insights into the Preference of Nairoviral DeISGylases for Interferon-Stimulated Gene Product 15 Originating from Certain Species. *J. Virol.* **2016**, *90*, 8314–8327. [CrossRef]
89. Campbell, J.B.; Buera, J.G. A comparison of the protective effect against Mengo virus infection in mice of interferons induced by polyI:C and Mengo virus. *Can. J. Microbiol.* **1971**, *17*, 1525–1532. [CrossRef]

90. Aznar, M.A.; Planelles, L.; Perez-Olivares, M.; Molina, C.; Garasa, S.; Etxeberría, I.; Perez, G.; Rodriguez, I.; Bolaños, E.; Lopez-Casas, P.; et al. Immunotherapeutic effects of intratumoral nanoplexed poly I:C. *J. Immunother. Cancer* **2019**, *7*, 116. [CrossRef]
91. Tong, J.; Zhu, C.; Lai, H.; Feng, C.; Zhou, D. Potent Neutralization Antibodies Induced by a Recombinant Trimeric Spike Protein Vaccine Candidate Containing PIKA Adjuvant for COVID-19. *Vaccines* **2021**, *9*, 296. [CrossRef]
92. Garg, R.; Latimer, L.; Gerdts, V.; Potter, A.; van Drunen Littel-van den Hurk, S. The respiratory syncytial virus fusion protein formulated with a novel combination adjuvant induces balanced immune responses in lambs with maternal antibodies. *Vaccine* **2015**, *33*, 1338–1344. [CrossRef] [PubMed]
93. Squillaro, T.; Peluso, G.; Galderisi, U. Clinical Trials With Mesenchymal Stem Cells: An Update. *Cell Transplant.* **2016**, *25*, 829–848. [CrossRef] [PubMed]
94. Raicevic, G.; Najar, M.; Busser, H.; Crompot, E.; Bron, D.; Toungouz, M.; Lagneaux, L. Comparison and immunobiological characterization of retinoic acid inducible gene-I-like receptor expression in mesenchymal stromal cells. *Sci. Rep.* **2017**, *7*, 2896. [CrossRef] [PubMed]
95. Song, N.; Scholtemeijer, M.; Shah, K. Mesenchymal Stem Cell Immunomodulation: Mechanisms and Therapeutic Potential. *Trends Pharmacol. Sci.* **2020**, *41*, 653–664. [CrossRef] [PubMed]
96. Shi, L.; Wang, L.; Xu, R.; Zhang, C.; Xie, Y.; Liu, K.; Li, T.; Hu, W.; Zhen, C.; Wang, F.-S. Mesenchymal stem cell therapy for severe COVID-19. *Signal Transduct. Target. Ther.* **2021**, *6*, 339. [CrossRef]
97. Sleem, A.; Saleh, F. Mesenchymal stem cells in the fight against viruses: Face to face with the invisible enemy. *Curr. Res. Transl. Med.* **2020**, *68*, 105–110. [CrossRef]
98. Gentile, P.; Sterodimas, A.; Pizzicannella, J.; Calabrese, C.; Garcovich, S. Research progress on Mesenchymal Stem Cells (MSCs), Adipose-Derived Mesenchymal Stem Cells (AD-MSCs), Drugs, and Vaccines in Inhibiting COVID-19 Disease. *Aging Dis.* **2020**, *11*, 1191–1201. [CrossRef]
99. Rossignol, J.-F.; Abu-Zekry, M.; Hussein, A.; Santoro, M.G. Effect of nitazoxanide for treatment of severe rotavirus diarrhoea: Randomised double-blind placebo-controlled trial. *Lancet* **2006**, *368*, 124–129. [CrossRef]
100. Haffizulla, J.; Hartman, A.; Hoppers, M.; Resnick, H.; Samudrala, S.; Ginocchio, C.; Bardin, M.; Rossignol, J.-F. Effect of nitazoxanide in adults and adolescents with acute uncomplicated influenza: A double-blind, randomised, placebo-controlled, phase 2b/3 trial. *Lancet Infect. Dis.* **2014**, *14*, 609–618. [CrossRef]
101. Jasenosky, L.D.; Cadena, C.; Mire, C.E.; Borisevich, V.; Haridas, V.; Ranjbar, S.; Nambu, A.; Bavari, S.; Soloveva, V.; Sadukhan, S.; et al. The FDA-Approved Oral Drug Nitazoxanide Amplifies Host Antiviral Responses and Inhibits Ebola Virus. *iScience* **2019**, *19*, 1279–1290. [CrossRef] [PubMed]
102. Rossignol, J.F.; El-Gohary, Y.M. Nitazoxanide in the treatment of viral gastroenteritis: A randomized double-blind placebo-controlled clinical trial. *Aliment. Pharmacol. Ther.* **2006**, *24*, 1423–1430. [CrossRef]
103. Wu, Z.; Graf, F.E.; Hirsch, H.H. Acitretin and Retinoic Acid Derivatives Inhibit BK Polyomavirus Replication in Primary Human Proximal Renal Tubular Epithelial and Urothelial Cells. *J. Virol.* **2021**, *95*, e00127-21. [CrossRef]
104. Li, P.; Kaiser, P.; Lampiris, H.W.; Kim, P.; Yukl, S.A.; Havlir, D.V.; Greene, W.C.; Wong, J.K. Stimulating the RIG-I pathway to kill cells in the latent HIV reservoir following viral reactivation. *Nat. Med.* **2016**, *22*, 807–811. [CrossRef] [PubMed]
105. Shin, D.S.; Han, S.S.; Kim, T.L.; Jang, J.W.; Seo, H.-M.; Kim, J.S. Treatment of Recalcitrant Viral Warts with Combination Therapy of Systemic Acitretin and Diphenylcyclopropenone Immunotherapy. *Ann. Dermatol.* **2020**, *32*, 243–246. [CrossRef] [PubMed]
106. Wang, H.; Ding, Y.; Zhou, J.; Sun, X.; Wang, S. The in vitro and in vivo antiviral effects of salidroside from *Rhodiola rosea* L. against coxsackievirus B3. *Phytomedicine* **2009**, *16*, 146–155. [CrossRef] [PubMed]
107. Sharma, N.; Mishra, K.P.; Ganju, L. Salidroside exhibits anti-dengue virus activity by upregulating host innate immune factors. *Arch. Virol.* **2016**, *161*, 3331–3344. [CrossRef]
108. Lu, R.; Wu, Y.; Guo, H.; Zhang, Z.; He, Y. Salidroside Protects Against Influenza A Virus-Induced Acute Lung Injury in Mice. *Dose Response* **2021**, *19*, 15593258211011335. [CrossRef]
109. Zhang, X.; Xie, L.; Long, J.; Xie, Q.; Zheng, Y.; Liu, K.; Li, X. Salidroside: A review of its recent advances in synthetic pathways and pharmacological properties. *Chem. Biol. Interact.* **2021**, *339*, 109268. [CrossRef]
110. Li, D.; Gale, R.P.; Liu, Y.; Lei, B.; Wang, Y.; Diao, D.; Zhang, M. 5′-Triphosphate siRNA targeting MDR1 reverses multi-drug resistance and activates RIG-I-induced immune-stimulatory and apoptotic effects against human myeloid leukaemia cells. *Leuk. Res.* **2017**, *58*, 23–30. [CrossRef]
111. Poeck, H.; Besch, R.; Maihoefer, C.; Renn, M.; Tormo, D.; Morskaya, S.S.; Kirschnek, S.; Gaffal, E.; Landsberg, J.; Hellmuth, J.; et al. 5′-Triphosphate-siRNA: Turning gene silencing and Rig-I activation against melanoma. *Nat. Med.* **2008**, *14*, 1256–1263. [CrossRef] [PubMed]
112. Chakravarthy, K.V.; Bonoiu, A.C.; Davis, W.G.; Ranjan, P.; Ding, H.; Hu, R.; Bowzard, J.B.; Bergey, E.J.; Katz, J.M.; Knight, P.R.; et al. Gold nanorod delivery of an ssRNA immune activator inhibits pandemic H1N1 influenza viral replication. *Proc. Natl. Acad. Sci. USA* **2010**, *107*, 10172–10177. [CrossRef] [PubMed]
113. Ho, V.; Yong, H.Y.; Chevrier, M.; Narang, V.; Lum, J.; Toh, Y.-X.; Lee, B.; Chen, J.; Tan, E.Y.; Luo, D.; et al. RIG-I Activation by a Designer Short RNA Ligand Protects Human Immune Cells against Dengue Virus Infection without Causing Cytotoxicity. *J. Virol.* **2019**, *93*, e00102-19. [CrossRef] [PubMed]

114. Mao, T.; Israelow, B.; Lucas, C.; Vogels, C.B.F.; Gomez-Calvo, M.L.; Fedorova, O.; Breban, M.I.; Menasche, B.L.; Dong, H.; Linehan, M.; et al. A stem-loop RNA RIG-I agonist protects against acute and chronic SARS-CoV-2 infection in mice. *J. Exp. Med.* **2022**, *219*, e20211818. [CrossRef] [PubMed]
115. Goulet, M.-L.; Olagnier, D.; Xu, Z.; Paz, S.; Belgnaoui, S.M.; Lafferty, E.I.; Janelle, V.; Arguello, M.; Paquet, M.; Ghneim, K.; et al. Systems analysis of a RIG-I agonist inducing broad spectrum inhibition of virus infectivity. *PLoS Pathog.* **2013**, *9*, e1003298. [CrossRef]
116. Franco, E.J.; Pires de Mello, C.P.; Brown, A.N. Antiviral Evaluation of UV-4B and Interferon-Alpha Combination Regimens against Dengue Virus. *Viruses* **2021**, *13*, 771. [CrossRef]
117. Ranoa, D.R.E.; Parekh, A.D.; Pitroda, S.P.; Huang, X.; Darga, T.; Wong, A.C.; Huang, L.; Andrade, J.; Staley, J.P.; Satoh, T.; et al. Cancer therapies activate RIG-I-like receptor pathway through endogenous non-coding RNAs. *Oncotarget* **2016**, *7*, 26496–26515. [CrossRef]
118. Wang, Z.; Chen, J.; Hu, J.; Zhang, H.; Xu, F.; He, W.; Wang, X.; Li, M.; Lu, W.; Zeng, G.; et al. cGAS/STING axis mediates a topoisomerase II inhibitor-induced tumor immunogenicity. *J. Clin. Investig.* **2019**, *129*, 4850–4862. [CrossRef]
119. Brzostek-Racine, S.; Gordon, C.; Van Scoy, S.; Reich, N.C. The DNA damage response induces IFN. *J. Immunol.* **2011**, *187*, 5336–5345. [CrossRef]
120. Zhu, S.; Waguespack, M.; Barker, S.A.; Li, S. Doxorubicin directs the accumulation of interleukin-12-induced IFNγ into tumors for enhancing STAT1 dependent antitumor effect. *Clin. Cancer Res.* **2007**, *13*, 4252–4260. [CrossRef]
121. Tesniere, A.; Schlemmer, F.; Boige, V.; Kepp, O.; Martins, I.; Ghiringhelli, F.; Aymeric, L.; Michaud, M.; Apetoh, L.; Barault, L.; et al. Immunogenic death of colon cancer cells treated with oxaliplatin. *Oncogene* **2010**, *29*, 482–491. [CrossRef] [PubMed]
122. Sadraeian, M.; Zhang, L.; Aavani, F.; Biazar, E.; Jin, D. Viral inactivation by light. *eLight* **2022**, *2*, 18. [CrossRef]
123. Kagan, A.B.; Garrison, D.A.; Anders, N.M.; Webster, J.A.; Baker, S.D.; Yegnasubramanian, S.; Rudek, M.A. DNA methyltransferase inhibitor exposure-response: Challenges and opportunities. *Clin. Transl. Sci.* **2023**, *16*, 1309–1322. [CrossRef]
124. Issa, J.-P. Optimizing therapy with methylation inhibitors in myelodysplastic syndromes: Dose, duration, and patient selection. *Nat. Clin. Pract. Oncol.* **2005**, *2* (Suppl. S1), S24–S29. [CrossRef] [PubMed]
125. Roulois, D.; Yau, H.L.; De Carvalho, D.D. Pharmacological DNA demethylation: Implications for cancer immunotherapy. *Oncoimmunology* **2016**, *5*, e1090077. [CrossRef] [PubMed]
126. Liu, X.; Zheng, F.; Tian, L.; Li, T.; Zhang, Z.; Ren, Z.; Chen, X.; Chen, W.; Li, K.; Sheng, J. Lidocaine inhibits influenza a virus replication by up-regulating IFNα4 via TBK1-IRF7 and JNK-AP1 signaling pathways. *Int. Immunopharmacol.* **2023**, *115*, 109706. [CrossRef]
127. Bedard, K.M.; Wang, M.L.; Proll, S.C.; Loo, Y.-M.; Katze, M.G.; Gale, M.; Iadonato, S.P. Isoflavone agonists of IRF-3 dependent signaling have antiviral activity against RNA viruses. *J. Virol.* **2012**, *86*, 7334–7344. [CrossRef]
128. Andres, A.; Donovan, S.M.; Kuhlenschmidt, M.S. Soy isoflavones and virus infections. *J. Nutr. Biochem.* **2009**, *20*, 563–569. [CrossRef]
129. Pattabhi, S.; Wilkins, C.R.; Dong, R.; Knoll, M.L.; Posakony, J.; Kaiser, S.; Mire, C.E.; Wang, M.L.; Ireton, R.C.; Geisbert, T.W.; et al. Targeting Innate Immunity for Antiviral Therapy through Small Molecule Agonists of the RLR Pathway. *J. Virol.* **2015**, *90*, 2372–2387. [CrossRef]
130. Huryn, D.M.; Kornfilt, D.J.P.; Wipf, P. p97: An Emerging Target for Cancer, Neurodegenerative Diseases, and Viral Infections. *J. Med. Chem.* **2020**, *63*, 1892–1907. [CrossRef]
131. Ye, Z.; Wang, K.; Chen, L.; Jin, X.; Chen, H.; Tang, G.; Yao, S.Q.; Feng, Z.; Zhang, C.-J. A targeted covalent inhibitor of p97 with proteome-wide selectivity. *Acta Pharm. Sin. B* **2022**, *12*, 982–989. [CrossRef] [PubMed]
132. Chisamore, M.J.; Cunningham, M.E.; Flores, O.; Wilkinson, H.A.; Chen, J.D. Characterization of a novel small molecule subtype specific estrogen-related receptor alpha antagonist in MCF-7 breast cancer cells. *PLoS ONE* **2009**, *4*, e5624. [CrossRef] [PubMed]
133. He, X.; Ma, S.; Tian, Y.; Wei, C.; Zhu, Y.; Li, F.; Zhang, P.; Wang, P.; Zhang, Y.; Zhong, H. ERRα negatively regulates type I interferon induction by inhibiting TBK1-IRF3 interaction. *PLoS Pathog.* **2017**, *13*, e1006347. [CrossRef] [PubMed]
134. Hwang, J.; Purdy, J.G.; Wu, K.; Rabinowitz, J.D.; Shenk, T. Estrogen-related receptor α is required for efficient human cytomegalovirus replication. *Proc. Natl. Acad. Sci. USA* **2014**, *111*, E5706–E5715. [CrossRef] [PubMed]
135. Karnati, K.R.; Wang, Y.; Du, Y. Exploring the binding mode and thermodynamics of inverse agonists against estrogen-related receptor alpha. *RSC Adv.* **2020**, *10*, 16659–16668. [CrossRef]
136. Lynch, C.; Zhao, J.; Sakamuru, S.; Zhang, L.; Huang, R.; Witt, K.L.; Merrick, B.A.; Teng, C.T.; Xia, M. Identification of Compounds That Inhibit Estrogen-Related Receptor Alpha Signaling Using High-Throughput Screening Assays. *Molecules* **2019**, *24*, 841. [CrossRef]
137. Wang, J.; Fang, F.; Huang, Z.; Wang, Y.; Wong, C. Kaempferol is an estrogen-related receptor alpha and gamma inverse agonist. *FEBS Lett.* **2009**, *583*, 643–647. [CrossRef]
138. Li, Q.; Wang, Y.; Zhang, L.; Chen, L.; Du, Y.; Ye, T.; Shi, X. Naringenin exerts anti-angiogenic effects in human endothelial cells: Involvement of ERRα/VEGF/KDR signaling pathway. *Fitoterapia* **2016**, *111*, 78–86. [CrossRef]
139. Ning, Y.; Chen, H.; Du, Y.; Ling, H.; Zhang, L.; Chen, L.; Qi, H.; Shi, X.; Li, Q. A novel compound LingH2-10 inhibits the growth of triple negative breast cancer cells in vitro and in vivo as a selective inverse agonist of estrogen-related receptor α. *Biomed. Pharmacother.* **2017**, *93*, 913–922. [CrossRef]

140. Duellman, S.J.; Calaoagan, J.M.; Sato, B.G.; Fine, R.; Klebansky, B.; Chao, W.-R.; Hobbs, P.; Collins, N.; Sambucetti, L.; Laderoute, K.R. A novel steroidal inhibitor of estrogen-related receptor α (ERRα). *Biochem. Pharmacol.* **2010**, *80*, 819–826. [CrossRef]
141. Seo, W.; Yoo, S.; Zhong, Y.; Lee, S.-H.; Woo, S.-Y.; Choi, H.-S.; Won, M.; Roh, T.; Jeon, S.M.; Kim, K.T.; et al. Targeting ERRα promotes cytotoxic effects against acute myeloid leukemia through suppressing mitochondrial oxidative phosphorylation. *J. Hematol. Oncol.* **2022**, *15*, 156. [CrossRef] [PubMed]
142. Boland, M.R.; Tatonetti, N.P. Investigation of 7-dehydrocholesterol reductase pathway to elucidate off-target prenatal effects of pharmaceuticals: A systematic review. *Pharmacogenom. J.* **2016**, *16*, 411–429. [CrossRef] [PubMed]
143. Korade, Z.; Heffer, M.; Mirnics, K. Medication effects on developmental sterol biosynthesis. *Mol. Psychiatry* **2022**, *27*, 490–501. [CrossRef] [PubMed]
144. Tallman, K.A.; Allen, L.B.; Klingelsmith, K.B.; Anderson, A.; Genaro-Mattos, T.C.; Mirnics, K.; Porter, N.A.; Korade, Z. Prescription Medications Alter Neuronal and Glial Cholesterol Synthesis. *ACS Chem. Neurosci.* **2021**, *12*, 735–745. [CrossRef]
145. Wang, K.; Zhang, J.; Yang, Y.; Si, Y.; Zhou, Z.; Zhu, X.; Wu, S.; Liu, H.; Zhang, H.; Zhang, L.; et al. STING strengthens host anti-hantaviral immunity through an interferon-independent pathway. *Virol. Sin.* **2023**, *38*, 568–584. [CrossRef]
146. Fawzy, I.O.; Negm, M.; Ahmed, R.; Esmat, G.; Hamdi, N.; Abdelaziz, A.I. Tamoxifen alleviates hepatitis C virus-induced inhibition of both toll-like receptor 7 and JAK-STAT signalling pathways in PBMCs of infected Egyptian females. *J. Viral Hepat.* **2012**, *19*, 854–861. [CrossRef]
147. Zu, S.; Luo, D.; Li, L.; Ye, Q.; Li, R.-T.; Wang, Y.; Gao, M.; Yang, H.; Deng, Y.-Q.; Cheng, G. Tamoxifen and clomiphene inhibit SARS-CoV-2 infection by suppressing viral entry. *Signal Transduct. Target. Ther.* **2021**, *6*, 435. [CrossRef]
148. Cham, L.B.; Friedrich, S.-K.; Adomati, T.; Bhat, H.; Schiller, M.; Bergerhausen, M.; Hamdan, T.; Li, F.; Machlah, Y.M.; Ali, M.; et al. Tamoxifen Protects from Vesicular Stomatitis Virus Infection. *Pharmaceuticals* **2019**, *12*, 142. [CrossRef]
149. Xiao, J.; Li, W.; Zheng, X.; Qi, L.; Wang, H.; Zhang, C.; Wan, X.; Zheng, Y.; Zhong, R.; Zhou, X.; et al. Targeting 7-Dehydrocholesterol Reductase Integrates Cholesterol Metabolism and IRF3 Activation to Eliminate Infection. *Immunity* **2020**, *52*, 109–122.e6. [CrossRef]
150. Xu, G.; Salen, G.; Shefer, S.; Ness, G.C.; Chen, T.S.; Zhao, Z.; Salen, L.; Tint, G.S. Treatment of the cholesterol biosynthetic defect in Smith-Lemli-Opitz syndrome reproduced in rats by BM 15.766. *Gastroenterology* **1995**, *109*, 1301–1307. [CrossRef]
151. Ahmed, C.M.I.; Dabelic, R.; Martin, J.P.; Jager, L.D.; Haider, S.M.; Johnson, H.M. Enhancement of antiviral immunity by small molecule antagonist of suppressor of cytokine signaling. *J. Immunol.* **2010**, *185*, 1103–1113. [CrossRef]
152. Frey, K.G.; Ahmed, C.M.I.; Dabelic, R.; Jager, L.D.; Noon-Song, E.N.; Haider, S.M.; Johnson, H.M.; Bigley, N.J. HSV-1-induced SOCS-1 expression in keratinocytes: Use of a SOCS-1 antagonist to block a novel mechanism of viral immune evasion. *J. Immunol.* **2009**, *183*, 1253–1262. [CrossRef] [PubMed]
153. Ahmed, C.M.; Dabelic, R.; Bedoya, S.K.; Larkin, J.; Johnson, H.M. A SOCS1/3 Antagonist Peptide Protects Mice Against Lethal Infection with Influenza A Virus. *Front. Immunol.* **2015**, *6*, 574. [CrossRef]
154. Johnson, H.M.; Lewin, A.S.; Ahmed, C.M. SOCS, Intrinsic Virulence Factors, and Treatment of COVID-19. *Front. Immunol.* **2020**, *11*, 582102. [CrossRef] [PubMed]
155. Schräder, T.; Dudek, S.E.; Schreiber, A.; Ehrhardt, C.; Planz, O.; Ludwig, S. The clinically approved MEK inhibitor Trametinib efficiently blocks influenza A virus propagation and cytokine expression. *Antivir. Res.* **2018**, *157*, 80–92. [CrossRef]
156. Baturcam, E.; Vollmer, S.; Schlüter, H.; Maciewicz, R.A.; Kurian, N.; Vaarala, O.; Ludwig, S.; Cunoosamy, D.M. MEK inhibition drives anti-viral defence in RV but not RSV challenged human airway epithelial cells through AKT/p70S6K/4E-BP1 signalling. *Cell Commun. Signal.* **2019**, *17*, 78. [CrossRef] [PubMed]
157. Sakai, T. "RB-reactivator screening" as a novel cell-based assay for discoveries of molecular targeting agents including the first-in-class MEK inhibitor trametinib (trade name: Mekinist). *Pharmacol. Ther.* **2022**, *236*, 108234. [CrossRef] [PubMed]
158. McMillen, C.M.; Beezhold, D.H.; Blachere, F.M.; Othumpangat, S.; Kashon, M.L.; Noti, J.D. Inhibition of influenza A virus matrix and nonstructural gene expression using RNA interference. *Virology* **2016**, *497*, 171–184. [CrossRef]
159. Karothia, D.; Dash, P.K.; Parida, M.; Bhagyawant, S.; Kumar, J.S. Inhibition of West Nile virus Replication by Bifunctional siRNA Targeting the NS2A and NS5 Conserved Region. *Curr. Gene Ther.* **2018**, *18*, 180–190. [CrossRef]
160. Shi, X.; Zhang, X.; Chang, Y.; Jiang, B.; Deng, R.; Wang, A.; Zhang, G. Nonstructural protein 11 (nsp11) of porcine reproductive and respiratory syndrome virus (PRRSV) promotes PRRSV infection in MARC-145 cells. *BMC Vet. Res.* **2016**, *12*, 90. [CrossRef]
161. Mahmoodur, R.; Ali, I.; Husnain, T.; Riazuddin, S. RNA interference: The story of gene silencing in plants and humans. *Biotechnol. Adv.* **2008**, *26*, 202–209. [CrossRef]
162. Friedrich, M.; Pfeifer, G.; Binder, S.; Aigner, A.; Vollmer Barbosa, P.; Makert, G.R.; Fertey, J.; Ulbert, S.; Bodem, J.; König, E.-M.; et al. Selection and Validation of siRNAs Preventing Uptake and Replication of SARS-CoV-2. *Front. Bioeng. Biotechnol.* **2022**, *10*, 801870. [CrossRef] [PubMed]
163. Sharifi, A.; Amanlou, A.; Moosavi-Movahedi, F.; Golestanian, S.; Amanlou, M. Tetracyclines as a potential antiviral therapy against Crimean Congo hemorrhagic fever virus: Docking and molecular dynamic studies. *Comput. Biol. Chem.* **2017**, *70*, 1–6. [CrossRef] [PubMed]
164. Baikerikar, S. Curcumin and Natural Derivatives Inhibit Ebola Viral Proteins: An In silico Approach. *Pharmacogn. Res.* **2017**, *9*, S15–S22. [CrossRef] [PubMed]
165. Jennings, M.R.; Parks, R.J. Curcumin as an Antiviral Agent. *Viruses* **2020**, *12*, 1242. [CrossRef]

166. Liu, C.-L.; Hung, H.-C.; Lo, S.-C.; Chiang, C.-H.; Chen, I.J.; Hsu, J.T.A.; Hou, M.-H. Using mutagenesis to explore conserved residues in the RNA-binding groove of influenza A virus nucleoprotein for antiviral drug development. *Sci. Rep.* **2016**, *6*, 21662. [CrossRef]
167. Terrier, O.; Dilly, S.; Pizzorno, A.; Chalupska, D.; Humpolickova, J.; Bouřa, E.; Berenbaum, F.; Quideau, S.; Lina, B.; Fève, B.; et al. Antiviral Properties of the NSAID Drug Naproxen Targeting the Nucleoprotein of SARS-CoV-2 Coronavirus. *Molecules* **2021**, *26*, 2593. [CrossRef]
168. Lejal, N.; Tarus, B.; Bouguyon, E.; Chenavas, S.; Bertho, N.; Delmas, B.; Ruigrok, R.W.H.; Di Primo, C.; Slama-Schwok, A. Structure-based discovery of the novel antiviral properties of naproxen against the nucleoprotein of influenza A virus. *Antimicrob. Agents Chemother.* **2013**, *57*, 2231–2242. [CrossRef]
169. Kakisaka, M.; Sasaki, Y.; Yamada, K.; Kondoh, Y.; Hikono, H.; Osada, H.; Tomii, K.; Saito, T.; Aida, Y. A Novel Antiviral Target Structure Involved in the RNA Binding, Dimerization, and Nuclear Export Functions of the Influenza A Virus Nucleoprotein. *PLoS Pathog.* **2015**, *11*, e1005062. [CrossRef]
170. Durymanova Ono, E.A.; Iamamoto, K.; Castilho, J.G.; Carnieli, P.; de Novaes Oliveira, R.; Achkar, S.M.; Carrieri, M.L.; Kotait, I.; Brandão, P.E. In vitro and in vivo inhibition of rabies virus replication by RNA interference. *Braz. J. Microbiol.* **2013**, *44*, 879–882. [CrossRef]
171. Nitschinsk, K.M.; Clarke, D.T.; Idris, A.; McMillan, N.A. RNAi Targeting of Human Metapneumovirus P and N Genes Inhibits Viral Growth. *Intervirology* **2018**, *61*, 149–154. [CrossRef] [PubMed]
172. Zhang, G.; Ng, F.; Chen, M. Short-hairpin RNAs delivered by recombinant adeno-associated virus inhibited the replication of influenza A viruses in vitro. *Virology* **2021**, *564*, 46–52. [CrossRef] [PubMed]
173. Teng, D.; Obika, S.; Ueda, K.; Honda, T. A Small Interfering RNA Cocktail Targeting the Nucleoprotein and Large Protein Genes Suppresses Borna Disease Virus Infection. *Front. Microbiol.* **2019**, *10*, 2781. [CrossRef]
174. Phuong, N.H.; Kwak, C.; Heo, C.-K.; Cho, E.W.; Yang, J.; Poo, H. Development and Characterization of Monoclonal Antibodies against Nucleoprotein for Diagnosis of Influenza A Virus. *J. Microbiol. Biotechnol.* **2018**, *28*, 809–815. [CrossRef]
175. Zhang, T.; Wang, T.-C.; Zhao, P.-S.; Liang, M.; Gao, Y.-W.; Yang, S.-T.; Qin, C.; Wang, C.-Y.; Xia, X.-Z. Antisense oligonucleotides targeting the RNA binding region of the NP gene inhibit replication of highly pathogenic avian influenza virus H5N1. *Int. Immunopharmacol.* **2011**, *11*, 2057–2061. [CrossRef] [PubMed]
176. Cao, J.; Dong, S.; Liu, Y.; Zhou, M.; Guo, J.; Jia, X.; Zhang, Y.; Hou, Y.; Tian, M.; Xiao, G.; et al. Screening and Identification of Lujo Virus Entry Inhibitors from an Food and Drug Administration-Approved Drugs Library. *Front. Microbiol.* **2021**, *12*, 793519. [CrossRef]
177. Bad'urová, L.; Polčicová, K.; Omasta, B.; Ovečková, I.; Kocianová, E.; Tomášková, J. 2-Deoxy-D-glucose inhibits lymphocytic choriomeningitis virus propagation by targeting glycoprotein N-glycosylation. *Virol. J.* **2023**, *20*, 108. [CrossRef]
178. Pająk, B.; Zieliński, R.; Manning, J.T.; Matejin, S.; Paessler, S.; Fokt, I.; Emmett, M.R.; Priebe, W. The Antiviral Effects of 2-Deoxy-D-glucose (2-DG), a Dual D-Glucose and D-Mannose Mimetic, against SARS-CoV-2 and Other Highly Pathogenic Viruses. *Molecules* **2022**, *27*, 5928. [CrossRef]
179. Rehwinkel, J.; Gack, M.U. RIG-I-like receptors: Their regulation and roles in RNA sensing. *Nat. Rev. Immunol.* **2020**, *20*, 537–551. [CrossRef]
180. Jiang, Y.; Zhang, H.; Wang, J.; Chen, J.; Guo, Z.; Liu, Y.; Hua, H. Exploiting RIG-I-like receptor pathway for cancer immunotherapy. *J. Hematol. Oncol.* **2023**, *16*, 8. [CrossRef]
181. Liu, Y.; Goulet, M.-L.; Sze, A.; Hadj, S.B.; Belgnaoui, S.M.; Lababidi, R.R.; Zheng, C.; Fritz, J.H.; Olagnier, D.; Lin, R. RIG-I-Mediated STING Upregulation Restricts Herpes Simplex Virus 1 Infection. *J. Virol.* **2016**, *90*, 9406–9419. [CrossRef] [PubMed]
182. Xiang, J.; Yang, Z.; Zhou, Q. Lidocaine relieves murine allergic rhinitis by regulating the NF-κB and p38 MAPK pathways. *Exp. Ther. Med.* **2022**, *23*, 193. [CrossRef]
183. Pilna, H.; Hajkova, V.; Knitlova, J.; Liskova, J.; Elsterova, J.; Melkova, Z. Vaccinia Virus Expressing Interferon Regulatory Factor 3 Induces Higher Protective Immune Responses against Lethal Poxvirus Challenge in Atopic Organism. *Viruses* **2021**, *13*, 1986. [CrossRef] [PubMed]
184. Durham, G.A.; Williams, J.J.L.; Nasim, M.T.; Palmer, T.M. Targeting SOCS Proteins to Control JAK-STAT Signalling in Disease. *Trends Pharmacol. Sci.* **2019**, *40*, 298–308. [CrossRef] [PubMed]
185. Banjan, B.; Krishnan, D.; Koshy, A.J.; Soman, S.; Leelamma, A.; Raju, R.; Revikumar, A. In-silico screening and identification of potential drug-like compounds for dengue-associated thrombocytopenia from Carica papaya leaf extracts. *J. Biomol. Struct. Dyn.* **2023**, *41*, 5963–5981. [CrossRef] [PubMed]
186. Qamar, M.T.U.; Mumtaz, A.; Naseem, R.; Ali, A.; Fatima, T.; Jabbar, T.; Ahmad, Z.; Ashfaq, U.A. Molecular Docking Based Screening of Plant Flavonoids as Dengue NS1 Inhibitors. *Bioinformation* **2014**, *10*, 460–465. [CrossRef]
187. Beatty, P.R.; Puerta-Guardo, H.; Killingbeck, S.S.; Glasner, D.R.; Hopkins, K.; Harris, E. Dengue virus NS1 triggers endothelial permeability and vascular leak that is prevented by NS1 vaccination. *Sci. Transl. Med.* **2015**, *7*, 304ra141. [CrossRef]
188. Henchal, E.A.; Henchal, L.S.; Schlesinger, J.J. Synergistic interactions of anti-NS1 monoclonal antibodies protect passively immunized mice from lethal challenge with dengue 2 virus. *J. Gen. Virol.* **1988**, *69 Pt 8*, 2101–2107. [CrossRef]
189. Lai, Y.-C.; Chuang, Y.-C.; Liu, C.-C.; Ho, T.-S.; Lin, Y.-S.; Anderson, R.; Yeh, T.-M. Antibodies against Modified NS1 Wing Domain Peptide Protect against Dengue Virus Infection. *Sci. Rep.* **2017**, *7*, 6975. [CrossRef]

190. Wu, S.-F.; Liao, C.-L.; Lin, Y.-L.; Yeh, C.-T.; Chen, L.-K.; Huang, Y.-F.; Chou, H.-Y.; Huang, J.-L.; Shaio, M.-F.; Sytwu, H.-K. Evaluation of protective efficacy and immune mechanisms of using a non-structural protein NS1 in DNA vaccine against dengue 2 virus in mice. *Vaccine* **2003**, *21*, 3919–3929. [CrossRef]
191. Schlesinger, J.J.; Brandriss, M.W.; Walsh, E.E. Protection of mice against dengue 2 virus encephalitis by immunization with the dengue 2 virus non-structural glycoprotein NS1. *J. Gen. Virol.* **1987**, *68 Pt 3*, 853–857. [CrossRef] [PubMed]
192. Scott, T.; Paweska, J.T.; Arbuthnot, P.; Weinberg, M.S. Pathogenic effects of Rift Valley fever virus NSs gene are alleviated in cultured cells by expressed antiviral short hairpin RNAs. *Antivir. Ther.* **2012**, *17*, 643–656. [CrossRef] [PubMed]
193. Soldan, S.S.; Plassmeyer, M.L.; Matukonis, M.K.; González-Scarano, F. La Crosse virus nonstructural protein NSs counteracts the effects of short interfering RNA. *J. Virol.* **2005**, *79*, 234–244. [CrossRef] [PubMed]
194. Hedil, M.; Kormelink, R. Viral RNA Silencing Suppression: The Enigma of Bunyavirus NSs Proteins. *Viruses* **2016**, *8*, 208. [CrossRef] [PubMed]
195. Lai, Y.; Yan, Y.; Liao, S.; Li, Y.; Ye, Y.; Liu, N.; Zhao, F.; Xu, P. 3D-quantitative structure-activity relationship and antiviral effects of curcumin derivatives as potent inhibitors of influenza H1N1 neuraminidase. *Arch. Pharm. Res.* **2020**, *43*, 489–502. [CrossRef]
196. Henrich, S.; Cameron, A.; Bourenkov, G.P.; Kiefersauer, R.; Huber, R.; Lindberg, I.; Bode, W.; Than, M.E. The crystal structure of the proprotein processing proteinase furin explains its stringent specificity. *Nat. Struct. Biol.* **2003**, *10*, 520–526. [CrossRef]
197. Yang, H.Y.; Zheng, N.Q.; Li, D.M.; Gu, L.; Peng, X.M. Entecavir combined with furin inhibitor simultaneously reduces hepatitis B virus replication and e antigen secretion. *Virol. J.* **2014**, *11*, 165. [CrossRef]
198. Rojek, J.M.; Pasqual, G.; Sanchez, A.B.; Nguyen, N.-T.; de la Torre, J.-C.; Kunz, S. Targeting the proteolytic processing of the viral glycoprotein precursor is a promising novel antiviral strategy against arenaviruses. *J. Virol.* **2010**, *84*, 573–584. [CrossRef]

Tropical Medicine and Infectious Disease

MDPI

Communication

Factors Contributing to In-Hospital Mortality in Dengue: Insights from National Surveillance Data in Mexico (2020–2024)

Eder Fernando Ríos-Bracamontes [1,†], Oliver Mendoza-Cano [2,†], Agustin Lugo-Radillo [3], Ana Daniela Ortega-Ramírez [4] and Efrén Murillo-Zamora [5,*]

1. Departamento de Medicina Interna, Hospital General de Zona No. 1, Instituto Mexicano del Seguro Social, Av. Lapislázuli 250, Villa de Álvarez 28984, Mexico
2. Facultad de Ingeniería Civil, Universidad de Colima, km. 9 Carretera Colima-Coquimatlán, Coquimatlán 28400, Mexico
3. CONAHCyT—Facultad de Medicina y Cirugía, Universidad Autónoma Benito Juárez de Oaxaca, Ex Hacienda Aguilera S/N, Carr. a San Felipe del Agua, Oaxaca 68020, Mexico
4. Facultad de Medicina, Universidad de Colima, Av. Universidad 333, Colima 28040, Mexico
5. Unidad de Investigación en Epidemiología Clínica, Instituto Mexicano del Seguro Social, Av. Lapislázuli 250, Villa de Álvarez 28984, Mexico

* Correspondence: efren.murilloza@imss.gob.mx

† These authors contributed equally to this work.

Abstract: This study aimed to identify the factors associated with all-cause in-hospital mortality in laboratory-confirmed dengue cases from 2020 to mid-2024. A nationwide retrospective cohort study was conducted in Mexico and data from 18,436 participants were analyzed. Risk ratios (RRs) and 95% confidence intervals (CIs), estimated using generalized linear regression models, were used to evaluate the factors associated with all-cause in-hospital mortality risk. The overall case–fatality rate was 17.5 per 1000. In the multiple model, compared to dengue virus (DENV) 1 infections, DENV-2 (RR = 1.81, 95% CI 1.15–2.86) and DENV-3 (RR = 1.87, 95% CI 1.19–2.92) were associated with increased mortality risk. Patient characteristics, such as increasing age (RR = 1.02, 95% CI 1.01–1.03), type 2 diabetes mellitus (RR = 2.07, 95% CI 1.45–2.96), and chronic kidney disease (RR = 3.35, 95% CI 2.03–5.51), were also associated with an increased risk of a fatal outcome. We documented the influence of both the virus and individual susceptibility on mortality risk, underscoring the need for a comprehensive public health strategy for dengue.

Keywords: dengue; dengue virus; hospital mortality; public health

1. Introduction

Dengue fever represents a public health challenge worldwide. The disease can manifest in a range of severities, from mild symptoms to severe and potentially fatal conditions. The factors associated with dengue fever severity and mortality risk are numerous and include host characteristics such as patient age, comorbid conditions, previous dengue virus (DENV) infections, and biochemical biomarkers [1]. In Mexico, by the end of 2022, the reemergence of DENV-3 infections was observed and differences in disease outcomes had been documented according to the identified serotype [2]. Understanding the factors contributing to mortality in dengue patients is crucial for improving clinical management and reducing death rates.

The epidemiological surveillance of dengue in Mexico is coordinated by a specialized sub-system within the National System for Epidemiological Surveillance (SINAVE). According to guidelines, patients with suspected dengue (fever and at least two of the following: nausea, rash, myalgia or arthralgia, headache or retro-ocular pain, petechiae or leukopenia) are registered in the web-based SINAVE [3]. All patients provide a venous blood sample; reverse-transcription polymerase chain reaction (RT-PCR) is performed within the first

5 days of symptom onset, and serological testing is conducted after 6 days [4]. Patients are followed until recovery or death.

This study aimed to identify the factors associated with all-cause in-hospital mortality in laboratory-positive dengue cases. By analyzing data from a national surveillance system spanning from 2020 to mid-2024, we sought to provide comprehensive insights into the epidemiological and clinical determinants of dengue-related mortality.

2. Materials and Methods

A nationwide retrospective cohort study was conducted in Mexico, including individuals who were hospitalized due to RT-PCR confirmed dengue. Eligible participants were those with symptom onset from 1 January 2020 to 3 June 2024 (spanning 1615 days) and were identified through the records of SINAVE [5]. Patients diagnosed through serological assays or those with missing DENV serotype data were excluded.

Demographic and clinical data, including the personal histories of non-communicable diseases, were collected from the audited surveillance system. Medical records and death certificates, when applicable, served as the primary data sources.

The main binary outcome was all-cause in-hospital mortality. We computed summary statistics, including case–fatality rate (CFR), and used generalized linear models with a binomial distribution and a log-link function to estimate risk ratios (RRs) and 95% confidence intervals (CIs) for the factors associated with an increased mortality risk. A multiple generalized linear model was constructed with dengue in-hospital fatal outcome (no/yes) as the dependent variable. The independent variables included were sex, age (years), identified DENV serotype, and preexisting comorbidities (no/yes), specifically type 2 diabetes mellitus, hypertensive disease, chronic kidney disease, and immunosuppression from any cause.

Since we analyzed publicly available anonymized data solely for academic purposes, ethics approval to conduct this research was waived.

3. Results

Data from 18,436 participants were analyzed, with 323 in-hospital deaths recorded, resulting in an overall in-hospital CFR of 17.5 per 1000. The CFRs by DENV serotype were 9.2, 19.8, 17.7, and 21.5 per 1000 for serotypes 1, 2, 3, and 4, respectively. Figure 1 illustrates patient enrollment by date of symptom onset and the distribution of DENV serotypes. DENV-3 peaked from the second trimester of 2023 through to the end of the study period and was identified in 47.8% of patients.

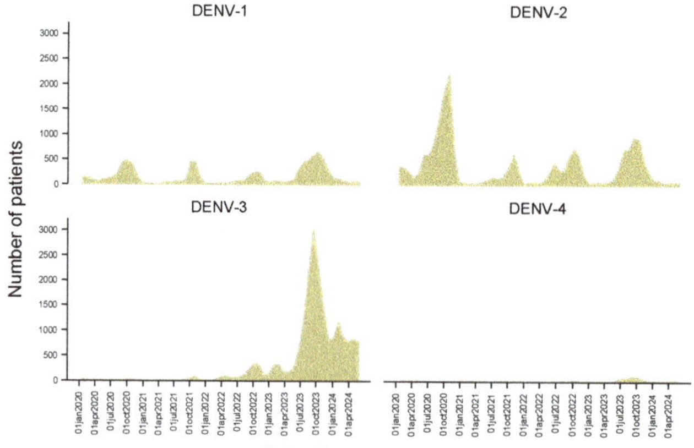

Figure 1. Date of symptom onset of the analyzed inpatients by identified dengue virus (DENV) serotype, Mexico 2020–2024. Note: The total number of patients by serotype was as follows: DENV-1, 2286 (12.4%); DENV-2, 7111 (38.6%); DENV-3, 8806 (47.8%); and DENV-4, 233 (1.3%).

Most participants were female (54.8%), with a mean age of 27.7 ± 17.6 years. Table 1 details the sample characteristics and in-hospital outcomes. Fatal cases were associated with older age (35.5 ± 25.4 vs. 24.5 ± 17.4 years, $p < 0.001$) and comorbidities such as type 2 diabetes mellitus, hypertensive disease, chronic kidney disease, and immunosuppression. The DENV serotype distribution varied significantly between fatal and non-fatal cases, with DENV-1 more common in non-fatal outcomes.

Table 1. Characteristics of the study sample for selected variables and in-hospital outcomes, Mexico 2020–2024.

Characteristic	Dengue Outcome		p
	Recovery (n = 18,113)	**Death (n = 323)**	
Sex			
Female	9923 (54.8)	170 (52.6)	0.441
Male	8190 (45.2)	153 (47.4)	
Age (mean ± SD, years)	24.5 ± 17.4	35.5 ± 25.4	<0.001
Age group (years)			
0–9	3098 (17.1)	53 (16.4)	<0.001
10–19	6098 (33.7)	66 (20.4)	
20–29	3407 (18.8)	39 (12.1)	
30–39	2154 (11.9)	35 (10.8)	
40–49	1407 (7.8)	32 (9.9)	
50–59	962 (5.3)	32 (9.9)	
60–69	580 (3.2)	24 (7.4)	
70 or above	407 (2.3)	42 (13.0)	
Isolated serotype			
DENV-1	2265 (12.5)	21 (6.5)	0.009
DENV-2	6970 (38.5)	141 (43.7)	
DENV-3	8650 (47.8)	156 (48.3)	
DENV-4	228 (1.3)	5 (1.6)	
Type 2 diabetes mellitus			
No	17,488 (96.6)	271 (83.9)	<0.001
Yes	625 (3.4)	52 (16.1)	
Hypertensive disease			
No	17,680 (97.6)	285 (88.2)	<0.001
Yes	433 (2.4)	38 (11.8)	
Chronic kidney disease			
No	18,030 (99.5)	307 (95.1)	<0.001
Yes	83 (0.5)	16 (4.9)	
Immunosuppression (any cause)			
No	18,074 (99.8)	320 (99.1)	0.008
Yes	39 (0.2)	3 (0.9)	

Abbreviations: SD, standard deviation; DENV, dengue virus. Notes: The p-value from ji-squared tests is presented, except if the mean and SD is specified, and there the t-test was used.

In the multiple generalized linear regression model (Table 2), DENV serotype was associated with in-hospital mortality risk. Compared to DENV-1 infection, DENV-2 was associated with an 81% increased risk (RR = 1.81, 95% CI 1.15–2.86, $p = 0.010$) and DENV-3 with an 87% increased risk (RR = 1.87, 95% CI 1.19–2.92, $p = 0.007$). The risk associated with DENV-4 was not statistically significant (RR = 1.88, 95% CI 0.73–4.86, $p = 0.190$).

Table 2. Factors associated with all-cause in-hospital mortality risk for dengue, Mexico 2020–2024.

	RR (95% CI), *p*	
	Bivariate Analysis	**Multiple Analysis**
Sex		
Female	1.00	1.00
Male	1.09 (0.88–1.35), 0.441	1.12 (0.90–1.39), 0.300
Age (years)	1.03 (1.02–1.04), <0.001	1.02 (1.01–1.03), <0.001
Isolated serotype		
DENV-1	1.00	1.00
DENV-2	2.16 (1.37–3.41), 0.001	1.81 (1.15–2.86), 0.010
DENV-3	1.93 (1.23–3.03), 0.005	1.87 (1.19–2.92), 0.007
DENV-4	2.34 (0.89–6.14), 0.085	1.88 (0.73–4.86), 0.190
Type 2 diabetes mellitus		
No	1.00	1.00
Yes	5.03 (3.78–6.70), <0.001	2.07 (1.45–2.96), <0.001
Hypertensive disease		
No	1.00	1.00
Yes	5.09 (3.67–7.04), <0.001	1.49 (0.99–2.23), 0.054
Chronic kidney disease		
No	1.00	1.00
Yes	9.65 (6.08–15.32), <0.001	3.35 (2.03–5.51), <0.001
Immunosuppression (any cause)		
No	1.00	1.00
Yes	4.11(1.37–12.28), 0.012	2.86 (0.99–8.29), 0.053

Abbreviations: RR, risk ratio; CI, confidence interval; DENV, dengue virus. Notes: (1) Log-binominal generalized linear regression models were employed to obtain RRs and 95% CIs; (2) Estimates from the multiple model were adjusted by all the variables listed in the table.

As shown in Table 2, each additional year in age was associated with a 2% increase in risk (RR = 1.02, 95% CI 1.01–1.03, $p < 0.001$). Chronic preexisting comorbidities were also significantly associated with mortality risk, including type 2 diabetes mellitus (RR = 2.07, 95% CI 1.45–2.96, $p < 0.001$) and chronic kidney disease (RR = 3.35, 95% CI 2.03–5.51, $p < 0.001$).

4. Discussion

Our results offer insights into the epidemiology and clinical determinants of in-hospital mortality among dengue patients. These findings underscore the need for effective management strategies to mitigate the mortality rates associated with this mosquito-borne disease [6].

The association between DENV serotype and mortality risk revealed that DENV-2 and DENV-3 infections were associated with an increased mortality risk compared to DENV-1. Some published studies have documented similar findings [7,8], while others have not observed differences in disease outcomes in terms of infectious serotype [9,10], highlighting the complexity and potential influence of other factors, such as regional variations, patient demographics, and coexisting medical conditions.

The temporal distribution of DENV serotypes, particularly the peak in DENV-3 cases during 2023, underscores the dynamic nature of dengue epidemiology [11]. This temporal variation may influence disease severity and should be considered in public health interventions aimed at controlling dengue outbreaks.

We also identified demographic and clinical factors associated with mortality risk. The presence of chronic comorbidities like type 2 diabetes mellitus and chronic kidney disease further increased mortality risk, underscoring the importance of managing these underlying health conditions in dengue patients to reduce adverse outcomes. Both conditions impose a substantial burden in Mexican adults [12,13].

The potential limitations of our study must be cited. Firstly, our use of data from an epidemiological surveillance system means that our findings are contingent upon the quality of this data, which introduces the potential for inherent biases or inaccuracies. Secondly, the scope of our study is constrained by the information collected within the epidemiological surveillance system under analysis. Clinical and epidemiological data, such as prior dengue episodes, are absent. A more comprehensive analysis, incorporating data from previous dengue fever episodes, could have strengthened our manuscript. Future research addressing this gap would be valuable from both public health and clinical viewpoints.

5. Conclusions

These results underscore the need for a comprehensive public health strategy for dengue. We documented the influence of both the virus and individual susceptibility on disease severity. Future research should confirm these findings in diverse populations and investigate the biological pathways leading to severe dengue.

Author Contributions: E.F.R.-B., O.M.-C. and E.M.-Z. conceptualized the research and developed the methodology. A.L.-R. and A.D.O.-R. developed the software and validated the results. E.F.R.-B. and O.M.-C. performed the formal analysis. A.D.O.-R. and E.M.-Z. conducted the investigation. Resources were provided by A.L.-R. E.M.-Z. managed data curation. E.F.R.-B., O.M.-C. and E.M.-Z. prepared the original draft. A.L.-R. and A.D.O.-R. contributed to reviewing and editing. E.M.-Z. handled data visualization. All authors have read and agreed to the published version of the manuscript.

Funding: This research received no external funding.

Institutional Review Board Statement: In this study, publicly available and fully deidentified data were analyzed solely for academic purposes. Therefore, approval from an ethics committee in health research was waived.

Informed Consent Statement: Patient consent was waived due to the fact the deidentified data were analyzed solely for academic purposes.

Data Availability Statement: The data presented in this study are publicly available and were provided by the General Directorate of Epidemiology of the Government of Mexico, which updates them on a weekly basis. The data can be accessed at the following link: https://www.gob.mx/salud/documentos/datos-abiertos-bases-historicas-de-enfermedades-transmitidas-por-vector (accessed on 21 July 2024).

Acknowledgments: The research group would like to thank the Health Research Coordination of the Mexican Institute of Social Security and the IMSS Foundation A.C. for their support in conducting and disseminating the results of this research.

Conflicts of Interest: The authors declare no conflicts of interest.

References

1. Tsheten, T.; Clements, A.C.A.; Gray, D.J.; Adhikary, R.K.; Furuya-Kanamori, L.; Wangdi, K. Clinical predictors of severe dengue: A systematic review and meta-analysis. *Infect. Dis. Poverty* **2021**, *10*, 123. [CrossRef] [PubMed]
2. Murugesan, A.; Manoharan, M. Dengue virus. In *Emerging and Reemerging Viral Pathogens*; Elsevier: Amsterdam, The Netherlands, 2020; pp. 281–359.
3. General Directorate of Epidemiology of the Government of Mexico. Manual of Standardized Procedures for the Epidemiological Surveillance of Vector-Borne Diseases. Available online: https://epidemiologia.salud.gob.mx/gobmx/salud/documentos/manuales/36_Manual_ETV.pdf (accessed on 2 August 2024). (In Spanish).
4. Institute of Epidemiological Diagnosis and Reference of the Government of Mexico. Guidelines for Laboratory Surveillance of Dengue and Other Arboviruses. Available online: https://www.gob.mx/cms/uploads/attachment/file/629265/Lineamientos_Dengue_Arb_V1-2021.pdf (accessed on 2 August 2024). (In Spanish).
5. General Directorate of Epidemiology of the Government of Mexico. Open Data: Vector-Borne Diseases (Dengue). Available online: https://www.gob.mx/salud/documentos/datos-abiertos-bases-historicas-de-enfermedades-transmitidas-por-vector (accessed on 21 July 2024). (In Spanish).
6. Das, P.R.; Khan, S.A.; Rahman, J.M.; Dewan, S.M.R. Effective Preventative Measures are Essential to Lower Disease Burden From Dengue and COVID-19 Co-infection in Bangladesh. *Environ. Health Insights* **2023**, *17*, 11786302231212774. [CrossRef] [PubMed]
7. Vicente, C.R.; Herbinger, K.H.; Froschl, G.; Malta Romano, C.; de Souza Areias Cabidelle, A.; Cerutti Junior, C. Serotype influences on dengue severity: A cross-sectional study on 485 confirmed dengue cases in Vitoria, Brazil. *BMC Infect. Dis.* **2016**, *16*, 320. [CrossRef] [PubMed]

8. Leng, X.Y.; Zhao, L.Z.; Liao, L.; Jin, K.H.; Feng, J.M.; Zhang, F.C. Genotype of dengue virus serotype 1 in relation to severe dengue in Guangzhou, China. *J. Med. Virol.* **2024**, *96*, e29635. [CrossRef] [PubMed]
9. Tsai, J.J.; Chang, K.; Chen, C.H.; Liao, C.L.; Chen, L.J.; Tsai, Y.Y.; Tsai, C.Y.; Lin, P.C.; Hsu, M.C.; Liu, L.T. Dengue virus serotype did not contribute to clinical severity or mortality in Taiwan's largest dengue outbreak in 2015. *Eur. J. Med. Res.* **2023**, *28*, 482. [CrossRef] [PubMed]
10. Quang Tran, K.; Hung Pham, V.; Thi Ngoc Tran, T.; Thao Mai, C.; Kieu Anh Pham, T.; Hoang Ngo, T.; Bui Thai Nguyen, H.; Manh Nguyen, C.; Van Duong, H.; Minh Nguyen, P. Dengue virus serotypes and related factors in children with dengue hemorrhagic fever in Southern Vietnam. *J. Infect. Dev. Ctries* **2024**, *18*, 495–500. [CrossRef] [PubMed]
11. Faridah, L.; Fauziah, N.; Agustian, D.; Mindra Jaya, I.G.N.; Eka Putra, R.; Ekawardhani, S.; Hidayath, N.; Damar Djati, I.; Carvajal, T.M.; Mayasari, W.; et al. Temporal Correlation Between Urban Microclimate, Vector Mosquito Abundance, and Dengue Cases. *J. Med. Entomol.* **2022**, *59*, 1008–1018. [CrossRef] [PubMed]
12. Antonio-Villa, N.E.; Bello-Chavolla, O.Y.; Fermin-Martinez, C.A.; Ramirez-Garcia, D.; Vargas-Vazquez, A.; Basile-Alvarez, M.R.; Nunez-Luna, A.; Sanchez-Castro, P.; Fernandez-Chirino, L.; Diaz-Sanchez, J.P.; et al. Diabetes subgroups and sociodemographic inequalities in Mexico: A cross-sectional analysis of nationally representative surveys from 2016 to 2022. *Lancet Reg. Health Am.* **2024**, *33*, 100732. [CrossRef] [PubMed]
13. Silva-Tinoco, R.; Cuatecontzi-Xochitiotzi, T.; Morales-Buenrostro, L.E.; Gracia-Ramos, A.E.; Aguilar-Salinas, C.A.; Castillo-Martinez, L. Prevalence of Chronic Kidney Disease in Individuals with Type 2 Diabetes Within Primary Care: A Cross-Sectional Study. *J. Prim. Care Community Health* **2024**, *15*, 21501319241259325. [CrossRef] [PubMed]

MDPI AG
Grosspeteranlage 5
4052 Basel
Switzerland
Tel.: +41 61 683 77 34

Tropical Medicine and Infectious Disease Editorial Office
E-mail: tropicalmed@mdpi.com
www.mdpi.com/journal/tropicalmed

www.ingramcontent.com/pod-product-compliance
Lightning Source LLC
Chambersburg PA
CBHW062100220926
51850CB00010B/2829
* 9 7 8 3 7 2 5 8 6 7 1 0 3 *